TAKE MY PROSTATE... PLEASE!

By Steve Bluestein

Published in the USA by:
BearManor Media
4700 Millenia Blvd.
Suite 175 PMB 90497
Orlando, FL 32839
www.bearmanormedia.com

Printed in the United States of America
ISBN   978-1-62933-492-9 (paperback)
          978-1-62933-493-6 (hardback)

Book and cover design by Darlene Swanson • www.van-garde.com

Dedication

I dedicate this book to Diane Nine, Bill Benbassat, Tom Blumenthal, Chris Beesemyer, Sue and Bill Gordon, Sue Kogen, Redenta Picazio, Bob Benjamin, Marlene and Bobby Badolato, Marlene Demko, Lillian Mizrah, Linda and Jay Wexler, Connie Kaplan, Deborah and Ryan Borchelt, Lynn Mitchell, Marilyn Michaels, Beverly Morganthal, Peter Fogel (So he won't whine), Cathy Ladman and Tom Frykman, Larry Feinberg, Bob Fisher of Los Angeles and Bob Fisher of Pennsylvania, Jon Stierwalt, Mike and Wendy Churukian, Jackie Jospeh, Mary Kennedy, Natalia Hunter, Kathryn Fenton, Lynne Turner, Brie Turner O'Banion, Jeanne Ardito, Adam Morra and Angela Abreu, Tanya Winston Martin, Paul and Meryl Lander, Elaine Good, Lloyd Silverman, Vicki Norris-Karten, Audrey Cohen, Mason Sommers, Rami Aizic, Richard Weinstein, Richard Gordon, Hadley Arnold, Bennet Yellin, Steve Tyler, Stuart Ross, Kevin Trudgeon, Mary Willard, Amy Goldberger, Janis Smythe, Cheryl Zicarro, Carol Morra, Randy Kirby, Paul Sanderson, Monica Flores, Sandra J. Mendelsohn Brown, Dr. Hyung Kim, Dr. Philip Yalowitz, Dr. Evan Koursh, Rich Ross, Linda Smisko, Katie Smisko, Sheila Washington, Lois Blake, Abby, Stuart and all the Wesslers, Susan Salter Roderick, Lynne Kuykendall, Jody and Andrew Colton, Karen Miller, Michael Mandell, Karen Alexander, Austin Brown,

Brian London, Dori Fram, Julie and Sam Bobrick, James Hornik and Ben Blake, who I could not have made it though without his continued support. The list could go on and on and on... if I have forgotten your name on this list please forgive me... I HAVE NO PROSTATE.

Oh yeah, and Monica Piper.

Preface

I have always been afraid that if I didn't worry about my health some horrible disease would kill me just as I was about to win the $300 million Lotto Jackpot. That would be my luck. I'm about to become a millionaire and die from a virus brought into the country by a flight attendant. As a child I didn't have the kind of parents who cared about nurturing. They were more into battling with each other than what their fights would do to their child—and what fights they were! I learned more four-letter words by the age of six than any child should be required to learn. I didn't know what a "bitch" was, but from my father's intonation I figured it wasn't good. I also learned at an early age that I had to look out for myself. That's how I lived my life: looking out for myself, which always meant worrying about my health. I can't tell you how many times I ran to the doctor for God-knows-what ailment that turned out to be nothing. I can't tell you how many scans and blood tests and X-rays and MRIs I've had only to be told there is nothing wrong with me. Can you believe it? Nothing wrong with me! I'm a crazy person, didn't they know that? Every one of the tests I took over the years came back negative. At one point I thought I was experiencing shortness of breath. I had a stress test. The doctor told me I had the heart of a twenty year old (I'm not doing the "So I should give it back" joke here. Thank you).

No matter what I thought was wrong with me, the doctors proved me wrong time and time again. It was always nothing despite the fact that I was sure it was life threatening. They began to use the word hypochondriac a lot when talking to me. I wasn't a hypochondriac. I truly wasn't. Then they began to use the words "get some help;" but I was getting some help. I was having blood tests and scans and examinations and… and… and…. Didn't they understand? I was being diligent about what could possibly be wrong with me. Oh wait, I get it now, not that kind of help. The sit-down-on-the-shrink's-couch-and-spill-your-guts-out kind of help. Been there. Done that. You can see how much good *that* did.

The anxiety these health issues caused me all through my twenties and thirties should have caused some damage to my health but it didn't. I was as healthy as a horse and my shrink told me so. He entered me in the Kentucky Derby. Yeah, that's right, I started seeing a shrink. I was having panic attacks. Even I recognized that having a panic attack at least once a week because you think you are dying is not normal. The shrink told me that my own mind was causing the symptoms I was experiencing. I had to realize the power of the human mind. I simply could not believe that I was manifesting these problems. Then he went into shrink high gear. He had me hold a ball suspended at the end of string. He told me to look at the ball and make it start rotating without moving my hand. I thought he was insane. How could I make the ball rotate? Suddenly it began to rotate. Then he told me to make the ball rotate in the other direction. Yeah, like that's gonna happen. Suddenly, the ball was rotating in the other direction. I looked at him in amazement because I had not consciously made the ball rotate or change directions. He told me *that's* how powerful the mind is. The mind can make you do and say and act in ways you have no control over, and that's why these symptoms keep coming up. I manifest them in my own mind because I'm so afraid I'm dying that my mind creates the symptoms to not make me wrong. This demonstration had a huge impact on me. It made me understand, for the first time, what was going on in my head and why I was always manifesting some kind of illness. Even with the knowledge of the power of the mind, I couldn't stop myself from seeing medical doctors for this ailment or that pain. What I paid in deductibles could have financed Trump's wall. I just didn't care; I was hell-bent on proving that I was ill or about to get ill or have been ill or should be ill because I had all these symptoms.

That's how my life went for decades—and then one day I got old. I got old and diagnosed with prostate cancer. I finally had what I had been worried about all my life. How I reacted and how I dealt with this medical emergency was strange even to me. All my friends were worried about me but not because I had cancer, because I was acting so normal. You see, what they didn't understand was it was almost a relief getting cancer. It was showing me that I wasn't wrong all those years. It just took me sixty years to prove myself right.

As I began the battle of fighting prostate cancer, the crazy stuff began to happen that only happens in my life. Things would go wrong, calls would be strange, people would be strange and finally there was the healing and getting back into my life. I observed it all like it wasn't happening to me. I sat back and watched all the insanity and saw the humor in everything. Being a comedian and a writer, I saw these mishaps as fodder for a new book. I decided to document my journey through prostate cancer, the surgery that followed, and finally the recovery. That's when I decided to write *Take My Prostate....* *Please!* It's a strange title, but it's almost what happened. When I found out I had cancer I was determined to have the prostate removed. I knew that if they removed the cancer my chances would be better at survival. I also knew that with my history, if they did not remove the prostate, every time I got an earache I would know that it was the cancer spreading. I wanted it out more for my peace of mind than for my protection from cancer. The doctors weren't so anxious to cut me open; they wanted to make sure I knew what I was getting myself into, and so we talked and talked and talked about all the various options. He told me I would probably outlive the cancer. He showed me the numbers but I didn't want to take that chance. I had finally had enough. In an attempt to be funny and to get him to do the surgery I just said to him, "Take my prostate.... Please!" He saw that I knew what I was getting into and he agreed. On the ride home from the doctor's office I thought, "What a great title for a book: *Take My Prostate.... Please!* Naturally I had to write it—and you just bought it.

(Just one tiny side note here: # 1) All through this book you will see side notes and numbers. Don't try to make sense of them. If it made any sense I'd still have my prostate and wouldn't have needed to write this book. Just enjoy the little joke and keep reading. Okay?

In The Beginning There Was A Neurotic Comedian

I was fine. For those of you who know me, you know those words never crossed my lips. "I am fine," was *not* part of my vocabulary. I was always a this hurts or that hurts kind of person. Yes, that was me, but, "I am fine," never! What the hell is fine? Fine is what other people are. I always had some kind of complaint—an ache, a pain, a cramp that came in the middle of the night to ruin my serenity. Here's the strange thing: I really was fine, and it was freaking me out. I had lived my entire life fearful that some illness would finally do me in. I believed that if I didn't watch out for illness and act upon it, I would die.

Where does that come from, you ask? I'll tell you. I had a mother who never wanted to admit her child was ever sick. She was the kind of mother that never should have been a mother. Her needs came first and her child's needs came second. If that child—namely me—got in the way of her needs, the child lost out. You see, a sick child was not on her schedule, and I paid the price for it. On the day I was rushed to the hospital with polio she told me there was nothing wrong with me. There was nothing wrong with me? I was in and out of a coma for a month. The paralysis made it impossible for me to bend from the waist up. I had spinal taps and so much blood-work done that I am still petrified of needles to this day. To my mother, there was nothing

1

wrong with me. Yep, just a little childhood polio is all I had. As suddenly as it came that's how suddenly it left—and with no side affects. Nothing is wrong with me? Nothing is wrong at all. Evidently my mother didn't get the how-to-be-a-mother handbook.

My polio episode taught me at an early age that if I didn't take care of myself, no one would. As I said before, I always felt that if I didn't worry about my health, something would get me. Some hideous disease would lie like a sleeping dragon in the depths of my immune system and would raise its ugly head to kill me with some kind of painful, extended illness that had no cure and wasn't covered by insurance. So, I worried. Fine? I was never fine. Even when I was fine, I wasn't fine. That's why as an adult I was always going to doctors just to make sure my "fine-o-meter" was working. I went to doctors like some people go to the movies. I had a punch card for my urologist. With each visit he'd punch a hole in the card and if I got ten holes punched, I got a free urinalysis.

One doctor actually said to me, "You have the heart of an athlete," and I thought to myself, *Sure, Roberto Clemente...he's dead.*

"So why do I pant when I run up the stairs?"

"Join a gym. Do more cardio," is all that doctor said.

In an effort to ward off any illness that could possibly get me, I joined a gym—which my doctor applauded as a good step forward. I should have made him pay the monthly dues. In any case, I went every day, seven days a week for over ten years. There is nothing compulsive about me... except my personality. Then one day I looked at those weights and thought to myself, *I can't,* and I never went back to the gym again. As diligent as I was about exercising, that's how much I couldn't get myself to go back to lift weights. I had exercised for ten years and it hadn't helped my paranoia. Now I was just worried I was going to have a stroke at the gym.

I did continue on with healthy living though. I watched my diet and never smoked and I had stopped doing drugs and drinking years ago. I'm sober over thirty-five years. I truly took care of myself because I knew no one else was going to—and my shrink was proud of me for that. Despite all this, nothing was changing in my life. I was still afraid I was dying, and it seemed I had reached as far as I could go with psychiatry, so the shrink and I parted ways. He went to his beach house that I paid for and I went to hell in a hand basket.

This neurotic behavior went on for years unchecked. I actually had a dear friend say to me, "Do you realize since I have known you, you told me you thought you have had MS, Cancer, Leukemia, Lou Gehrig's disease, a stroke, arteriosclerosis, rosacea, psoriasis and crabs?" The sad part is, he was right. I did think I had all those things. I knew I had a problem and should be doing something about it. When I turned sixty I began to slow down and I tried to get the neurotic behavior under control. I realized that I was older now and nothing had killed me up to this point, so it was time to enjoy what I had left of my life.

I retired from show business from being an opening act for people like Donna Summer, Barry Manilow, Melissa Manchester, Frankie Valli, and a host of other big-name celebrities. I had worked on some of the greatest stages in Las Vegas, Reno, and Tahoe; but I was tired of the road. Tired of the travel. I was just tired. I got off the road and thought I was about to relax and enjoy the fruits of my labor... but those headaches, those headaches would not go away. Here's the hard part about being a hypochondriac: you never truly know when you are sick. I always had an internal battle—should I go to the doctor, should I not go to the doctor? It took a friend to say, "Go to the Goddamn doctor. He'll tell you there is nothing wrong with you and you can finally relax."

Off to the doctors I went once again. I knew in my heart of hearts that, like before, there would be nothing wrong. That's when life throws you a curve ball. My blood pressure was stroke level. You know your blood pressure is high when the nurse looks at the monitor, opens the exam room door, then yells down the hall, "HELEN!!! Come in here you won't believe this!"

I was immediately put on pills and monitored until they could get my blood pressure down to a normal level. My reaction to all of this was a surprise to everyone—myself included. I wasn't afraid I was going to die. I just did what the doctor ordered and never mentioned my medical condition again. I didn't panic. I didn't obsess. I simply did what had to be done. It's a strange thing, this mind of mine. It's like it was saying, "See, I told you, you were sick." It was like this high blood pressure was proof that what I had been worrying about for all those years was real. I was validated. I wasn't crazy—I was actually sick.

This little blood pressure episode was a harbinger of things to come. It wasn't my mind that was making me sick. It was my age. It took sixty years, but the illnesses finally started showing up. I guess I showed that shrink a thing or two. I knew what to worry about. Then the biggest event of my life happened: I fell down a flight of stairs. I fell in my own house. I couldn't even sue anyone because it was my own house. I broke two ribs and was left with a constant pain in my left shoulder blade. The tests and pain meds and injections did nothing for the pain. Finally I had yet another MRI, and this time it revealed I had a ruptured disc in my neck caused by the fall. I needed surgery to cure it. That was my very first real surgery (unless you count a few nose jobs) to repair the ruptured disc. In doing the blood work for the pre-surgery workup, they found blood in my urine. They wanted to do a cystoscopy to see what it was. I said, "Sure, no problem." Nothing had ever been wrong with me even though I feared it had been my whole life. No test had ever come back with a bad result, so I wasn't worried. Until I got the phone call.

"Steve, that thing we took out of your bladder was cancer. You have bladder cancer."

The one thing I had feared and worried about my entire life was here, and when the doctor told me my diagnosis once again, I was as calm as could be. Too calm, it turns out. He called back an hour later. He was worried that my quiet response to the news was shock and that I was freaking out by now. "Listen, you have cancer but it's the best cancer you can get. Stage one. Non-invasive. No chemo. No radiation. You're just going to need a cystoscopy for the next six years every three months, then every six months then once a year until we are sure it has not returned."

That's what I did. After I had my disc surgery I started monitoring my bladder cancer and had those cystoscopies every time they were due. It was like I belonged to religious cult, "Our Lady of the Probing Penis." I saw my doctor more than Cher sees her plastic surgeon. It was like we were dating—without the sex, cohabitation, or joint checking account.

I made it my responsibility to make sure my health was always a top priority. I had an annual check-up like some people go on vacation. Once a year I went in for a check-up just to make sure nothing had returned or mutated or fallen off, and of course I had my annual cystoscopy. I would tell my friends, "I'm going in for the fifty-thousand mile check-up and to have my tires rotated." To me, everything was a joke.

In case you're wondering what a cystoscopy is, it's a lot of fun. You lie on a table spread-eagle with two female nurses standing and staring at your crotch as your man-parts hang out there like the American flag over the Super Bowl. The doctor shoves a probe up your shavantz so he can see inside your bladder. At one of these appointments the doctor said to me, "Want to see yourself on TV?" (The monitor they use to look inside the bladder).

I said, "No thanks. I've seen myself on TV. If Oprah is in there let me know, then I'll look."

I love this doctor. He is the parent I never had. He cares about me, so when I go to see him it's with mixed emotions. He's like a parent you have to pay to love you. Wait. That is *just* like my real parents. When the doctor asked on this last visit, "Any complaints?" my answer was, "Not a one." This made him very suspicious. I've been going to him for years. There was always a complaint. If I didn't have a complaint this time, it's either Alzheimer's or a brain tumor. Suddenly he's typing very quickly into the computer chart. He pokes me here. He pushes me there. We never make eye contact because he's afraid he's found something.

"The nurse will take your vitals and blood," he says like a fatherly Count Dracula. We shake. I ask him what he's doing for Thanksgiving. He tells me he's having a huge dinner party with friends and family and then he doesn't invite me—just like my real parents!

I leave his office knowing that I am good-to-go. Why? I have no complaints because I am fine. The next day the phone rings.

"Steve? It's Dr. Yalowitz. Listen, your blood pressure is sky-high again, and your PSA is slightly elevated."

I asked him if he had the right chart because, "I am fine."

He assured me he did. My blood pressure was 180 over 116. Normal blood pressure is 120 over 80. It's been an ongoing struggle for me with this blood pressure over the years. It's hard to control even with the meds. Now about the PSA test. PSA is the test they use to determine if there is cancer cells in your prostate. Mine was slightly higher than it had been the last time I took the test. It was now 6.5. Now, 6.5 is not astronomical but when it jumps from 4.8 to 6.5 in six months, that throws up a red flag. He's wants me to see a specialist. I am so glad I asked for that second test when I came in this time.

Flash forward ten days. There I am on the specialist's table splayed open again like a filet of flounder at Bubba Gump Shrimp Company. "We need to do a biopsy," the specialist says with the concern of Dr. Demento.

Oh great. I'm going to be skewered like a barbecue chicken, only with anesthesia instead of barbecue sauce, is all I can think of. My mind is in overdrive. I keep thinking of only the worst, *a biopsy? Isn't that where they find the tumor and tell you to make final arrangements?* When I am faced with this kind of life-threatening situation is when my grandmother's negativity raises its ugly head. She could take any situation and make it worse, "Ya know who died? Sylvia. She went in for a simple D&C and right in the middle of the procedure she stroked. There she was dead on the table while her family was in the cafeteria having soup. Happens more than you care to think about. More chicken?"

Those are the thoughts I'm bringing with me to the biopsy. For those of you who have never had a prostate biopsy, let me give you a rundown of how it plays out. First you strip from the waist down— and not like you did on a date in the back seat of your father's car. Then some nameless technician asks you to lie on your side. You do. I looked over my shoulder and see the nurse coming towards me with something that looks like a metal dildo the size of a drainpipe covered in a prophylactic. She tells me to look at the wall. I don't know why, but I do. Suddenly I am being butt-fucked by a complete stranger and without dinner and movie first.

As I'm lying there, I turn my head over my shoulder and say to the twenty-two year old nurse, "This was a childhood dream of yours, wasn't it?" I'm trying to make light of the situation. I'm a comedian. I'm trying to make her laugh. What I get from her is nothing—not even a smile. Now the specialist comes in with yet another specialist. To me, this is not a good sign. He needs a consultant to look up my ass? How much is this going to cost me? The two of them are now rummaging through my rectum like a pair of raccoons at a garbage dump. They need to take samples of the prostate. They do it by snipping little pieces out. I joke, "Leave some for me fellas," as they snap, snap, snip, snip. Done.

The last thing the doctor says to me as he takes my arm and walks me to the lobby, "Don't worry Steve, we got it very early."

"What? What did we get early?"

What a strange thing to say to a neurotic, I thought to myself as I walked into the lobby. I see other men sitting there waiting for their prostate biopsy. I want to scream to them, "Go back! It's a cookbook!" But I don't. I shake the doctor's hand and head home to wait for the results.

The very next day there was not a word from the doctor. Going under the assumption that no news is good news I was thrilled and continue on with my carefree life. Then I notice I have no Wi-Fi in my house. I run up to my home office and switch on the light. Nothing. The computer? Dead. The hall light is dead. I see a pattern forming. I had no electricity to the entire top floor of my house. The phone modem was there and then I realize my phone lines are dead. I still didn't worry—if there was anything important he would email me. Oh wait! No electricity, no computer, no phone, no lights, *no email!* I'm screwed. $400 later the electrician told me a plug in my guest room had shorted out and that's why the doctor couldn't call to tell me I was about to die. It's like the universe is preparing me for the next six months. It's the omen.

It must have been twenty minutes after the lights went back on when the phone rang. "I've been trying to reach you all day. The line has been busy, who have you been talking to?" says the panicked doctor.

"I know, I know, my electricity has been off. It's been hell over here" I half-laughingly get out.

He laughs too. It was the nervous laugh someone has when they have something to tell you but they don't want to tell it to you because it's bad news. "I knew you'd want to get the results," he continues on.

"Yeah, that would be nice. How long do I have?" I say, panicked like Little Eva on the railroad tracks.

"You have prostate cancer."

I hear the words and my world stops. I'm waiting for the musical punctuation of his sentence—you know like they do in the movies when they have come to an important plot point. It's usually followed by a choir of angels singing "Sweet Low Sweet Chariot." I get nothing. There was no sound. There was no cold or hot. I was just numb. In my head I am well aware that if a man lives long enough, at some point he will develop cancer in his prostate. Who knew I had lived long enough? Didn't seem long enough to me. In most cases, the cancer is slow-growing and the man will outlive it. But it is cancer, and when it happens to you and you hear those words, you suddenly do a quick inventory of your life. *Where did it go? How can I have lived long enough to have prostate cancer?*

The doctor breaks the silence, "We have to do something immediately."

We? We have to do something? I think it's my prostate on the chopping block here. I think *I* have to do something, but what do I do? Where do I go? Who do I call?

I lived in fear of the words, "You have cancer," all my life and now there they were. I didn't know what to do with them. How did I react? Strangely enough, after I got off the phone with the doctor, I broke out of my coma and sprung into action. No one was more surprised than I was. Instead of curling up in a ball and reviewing my will, I began making a plan. *Okay, let's get going,* was all I could think of. I was ready to fight this battle—however the medical profession was not. Let me tell you something about doctors' offices and that girl they pay $10 an hour to make appointments: there is no "immediately" in their world. STAT is just something that writers put into scripts of *Chicago Hope.* I tell her I must see the doctor immediately, she tells me the earliest she can get me in is three weeks. Three weeks! I've got cancer racing through my body and she wants me to wait *three weeks.* I beg, I plead, I all but cry. She has two people on hold, "Do you want that appointment or not? I can put you on the wait list in case someone dies...ah... cancels."

Why don't you just throw gasoline on my anxiety, lady? But what can I do? They have you over a barrel. I take the appointment in three weeks and hope I don't die in the meantime.

When I get off the phone my initial reaction to the three-week wait was good. During the day, my inner dialogue is, *Okay. We got it early. I'll be fine. Three weeks isn't that long to wait. What are you so worried about?* Here's my nighttime falling asleep inner dialogue: *What if it's spread to the lining of the pancreas? Maybe it's in my lungs now. I coughed this afternoon. Maybe I have lung cancer. What's this pain in the back of my head? Oh my God I've got cancer all over my body.* By then it's 4 a.m. and I can't fall back to sleep, so I walk around the house wondering who is going to pack up all this crap after I die. Now my anxiety kicks into high gear and I'm looking up movers and estate attorneys and mortuaries and…and… and… it's five o'clock in the morning. Even my dog thinks I'm insane as he sits there licking his balls.

The three weeks fly by like I've been stretched out on one of those medieval contraptions they use to pull arms and legs off criminals. The agony of the wait was unbearable. Why is it when you're on vacation in Europe three weeks fly by like it's ten minutes, but when you're waiting for something like an appointment to find out if your cancer has spread, the time feels like an eternity? In any case, I decided to see two doctors; a primary and another to get a second opinion. I see the primary on Monday and then have to pay for parking again on Tuesday for the second opinion because the son of a bitch appointment maker couldn't book me in on the same day to see both doctors despite the fact that are both in the same building. Ugh! Here's a question: doctors make six figures a year, some make seven figures a year. Would it kill them to validate my parking? How much of a hit to their income could it be? What would it mean, one less round of golf? We're paying $500 for an office visit and we have to pay for our own parking? Somewhere there is a karma button those doctors are going to get hit with when they waltz through the pearly gates…of hell.

When I finally get in to see the primary doctor I am greeted with "Why are you here?"

It's a good question. "Why am I here?" I should be in the south of France having drinks with writer-producer Kevin Rooney, but, "Prostate cancer," is all I managed to get out.

"No! How did you get that?"

I wanted to smack him in the face with my biopsy report. He

went to medical school and he's asking me how I got prostate cancer? Was he absent that day? Did he fail the cancer quiz? I keep my mouth shut and joke, "Well, if I knew that I would be in the south of France having drinks with Kevin Rooney."

He has no idea who this Emmy Award-winning writer is as he looks at the chart. He doesn't ask me to take off my clothes. He just goes into his caring loving speech that isn't caring or loving or a speech at all. It's just the talk he's given ten thousand times, "Look, at your age I can't guarantee you'll have an erection again. You're going to be incontinent for about two years and you will probably have erectile dysfunction for the rest of your life." This was the good news in his compassionate oration. Remind me not to invite him to my Christmas party. This guy has the bedside manner of Goebbels. Then he goes on, "See my nurse, let's make a date for the surgery. You'll need blah, blah, blah, blah..."

In my head I'm still in the south of France but Kevin Rooney has left the bar by now and I'm alone wondering why I feel like the world has left me to battle this all by myself. We end the interview. Oh yes, it was an interview. I was interviewing this doctor to see if I wanted him to do the surgery. I didn't.

Next day I see the second doctor for the second opinion. It's another $10 parking fee. As you can tell, I have this thing about doctors not validating parking. The doctor comes in, sits down and looks me in the eye.

"Let's discuss exactly what you're going to go through and what your options are." He then presents me flow charts and diagrams and he's drawing on that paper covering that's on every exam table in every doctor's exam room in the United States and he tells me percentages and reasons for this and reasons for that. I listen closely. I know that I may outlive this cancer, but I also know that with my personality, every time I get a pain someplace I'll know it's the cancer. I want this thing taken out. When it's out it will lessen my level of anxiety. I tell this to the doctor and it's then I make my little, "Take my prostate, please!" joke. He takes a minute to ponder what I've just told him, and then he agrees.

I love this guy! I feel protected. I feel safe. I feel his practice will take my insurance, and with my supplemental, I'll end up paying nothing. Okay, I've made up my mind. For this guy I'll pay for my own parking. This guy has compassion. This guy feels for what I'm about to go through. This guy is a winner! I'm going with the second opinion doctor. Done.

The doctor shakes my hands and tells me his surgical scheduler will come in and find a date for me. He has a matchmaker on staff? No you idiot, she's going to get me a surgical date and she is as sweet as pie. Sure she's sweet as pie, she has to be. She's going in for the kill. This is the woman who makes the big bucks for the doctor. If I book a surgery, he gets a salary. If he gets a salary, she gets a salary. This woman is smooth as silk as she weaves her web of open surgery dates and post-op appointment times.

"The doctor is very busy. He's out of town October second to the twentieth. He can't do it on the first and he's leaving town the first two weeks in November. What date would you like?"

I said, "Is he booked forty-five years from now?"

She giggles. We agree on a date in three weeks. The only open date left on his calendar. It's a good date—and when I say good date I say it with as much sarcasm as I can muster. It's a date that will interfere with everything on my schedule for the next three months; the show in Palm Springs I'm presently in, the annual event I do downtown, Thanksgiving, my early Christmas shopping, Christmas, New Years. Yep, I got a date that will just about ruin the entire fall season for me—but what are my choices? If I don't take the date in October, then I'll be recuperating right in the middle of Thanksgiving, Christmas, and New Years. Try and get someone to help you during that period—you can't—so I go for the earliest possible date I can get. There is one thing I am learning from this whole experience: cancer never comes at a convenient time.

I think I'm done. I have a date; what else is there to do? Turns out, lots. I am given a packet of chores I need to do in the next two weeks prior to surgery. Eisenhower didn't have this many plans when he invaded Europe. I need a colonoscopy, I need another cystoscopy, I need a chest X-ray, I need surgical clearance, I need an EKG. The only thing I didn't need was a note from my mother—good thing, she's been dead for two years. There was one more little thing to ensure my misery: my meds are not covered by insurance and they are $6,800 for a three-month supply. Did I forget anything? Oh yes... just shoot me now!

I Gave Elon Musk the Finger

I start on the list the doctor has given me. First thing on the agenda is a 10:30 a.m. appointment with a blood pressure doctor. Before I can have my surgery I need to get my blood pressure under control. This blood pressure thing has been a battle, and now I am about to see a blood pressure specialist. I often wonder how doctors chose their field of endeavor. I mean, what makes you decide you want to be a blood pressure specialist? Do they suddenly at the age of seven decide they have an affinity for the blood pressure cuff? These are the important questions that are running through my mind as I'm pulling out of the garage and heading for the appointment. My mind is always going like that. I am always writing some comedy bit. Suddenly a light comes on the dashboard of my new Tesla. That is correct. I bought a Tesla. If cancer is going to take my life at least I can have a car that will drive itself to the funeral. What is this message on a new car? "Right front tire needs air." This really pisses me off because I just put air in the left front tire last week. I had my crappy little Toyota for nine years. I never had to put air in the tires. I never had to put anything into it at all but gas. Now that I am a big-shot in the fancy new Tesla and I am putting air in the tires every other week. Oh well, these are the problems some people would love to have. I cannot complain because I need air in the tire of my Tesla.

There are people starving in the world. I am a horrible, selfish person to be upset about something like this with all that is going on in the world. Besides, I'll get the air in my tire later.

I see the doctor, and with the meds she ordered prior to today's visit, my blood pressure is now 117/77 controlled and she is thrilled. She clears me for surgery. However, she notices that my cancer doctor has prescribed a pill that's the same as that my kidney doctor prescribed. I have more doctors than the cast of *Grey's Anatomy*. She tells me she'll contact my cancer doctor and work it all out. I am free to go. As I'm walking out through the lobby I ask the receptionist cautiously, "So, do you guys validate parking?" She shakes her head no. I've found another doctor that does not validate parking. By this time I am used to the fact that no doctor in LA validates parking and I just head downstairs and pay the parking guy with a forced smile on my face.

After I leave the blood pressure doctor's office I begin my adventure to get air in my tire. I know there's a gas station on Wilshire. I head down Wilshire Blvd. It is bumper to bumper traffic, a virtual parking lot through Beverly Hills. A fifteen-minute drive has now taken me thirty minutes. The gas station is coming up on my left but I cannot get to the gas station due to subway construction on Wilshire. I can't turn left into the only gas station in Beverly Hills. I think the next one is in Oklahoma. We have not had a subway system in Los Angeles in 150 years. Today they decide to build one and block every street on my route to get air in my tires. So I go to the next light and turn left. I drive to Santa Monica Blvd because I know there are gas stations there. I pull into the first gas station I see. There is a big sign on the air pump, "OUT OF ORDER." To make matters worse, a truck has pulled in behind me and there is another truck servicing the pump in front of me. I'm trapped in a no-mans land of vehicle obstruction for twenty minutes while these giants of industry decide which gas pump they should block next. Does anyone see the irony here? I am in an electric car trapped at a gas station. Believe me I got some weird looks, "What the hell is he doing here? Did he pull in just so he could rub it in our faces? Get out of here you electric car freak!" I have a vivid imagination.

When the brain trust of truck drivers finally frees me I head to the next gas station. I drive all around the station looking for the air pump but the gas station doesn't have an air pump. Of all the gas stations on Santa Monica Blvd., I find the one station that decided that having an air pump would be too costly for them to install. What kind of gas station does not have an air pump? They have a mini-mart where you can get enough food to host twelve for Thanksgiving. You can get a Slurpee, a hotdog, a burrito, nachos, and a pizza, but you cannot get air for your tires. You can buy a lotto ticket, get milk and breath mints, but you cannot get air for your tires. At this gas station you can get anything you ever wanted if you were stranded on a desert island. I wonder, *Can I get prostate surgery here?* Then I realize this is all the prostate cancer's fault. If I had not gone to the doctor, I would not be on this journey. It is another reason I give myself to hate the cancer.

At this point I am frustrated and anxious and furious with anyone who has ever gotten air in their tires in the last decade. I think to myself, *Forget it. I'll get it done tomorrow.* I'm already an hour and a half into this drama and it is not helping my blood pressure. As I leave the gas station, I look down on the dashboard, and the warning light goes out. As suddenly as the light came on, it went off. How does this happen? How does a car need air in a tire, you don't put any air in, and suddenly it no longer needs air? Is there an air fairy that comes and fills your tires when you are not looking? I swear to you

I heard the car giggle as I went into my hissy fit. My only revenge, I scream, "Bite me, Elon Musk!"

In the meantime, the blood pressure doctor calls me on my cell, "Okay, I worked it out with your cancer doctor. Stop taking this med, start taking that med... put this med in a bottle... don't take that med... but make sure you take the med that is supposed to take..."

My ears start to bleed. "Can't you just send me this in an email?"

She agrees to email me and I'm back in bumper-to-bumper traffic in the city of angels. It appears that someone found a street in Los Angeles that hasn't been dug up yet and they have decided to dig it up, so I will not be able to get home until I am a guest in assisted living.

I get home and the blood pressure doctor has sent me the email message. I try to open it. It won't open. At this point I am positive that there is some kind of karma thing happening and I am being paid back for something I did to some comedy club owner in the 1980s. I gather my strength and I call tech support for Cedars Sinai hospital web site. I have never met a larger group of idiots. Not a single person can help me open the email. I ask to speak to a supervisor. He's dumber than the guy I just spoke to and gives me a Help Desk number. I call it. It's for employees. I email the blood pressure doctor, "Just send me the information via unsecured email before I have a stroke." I reasoned if unsecured emails were good enough for Hillary Clinton it should be good enough for me. I'm waiting for the doctor's email. I take my blood pressure; it's like five million over two thousand. I get the email from the doctor and the medication problem is solved. I move on to the next item on the list my surgeon has given me.

I'm going to need another cystoscopy. I'm not happy about this on a good day, but when you learned you've got cancer, it opens up a whole world of paranoia. *The prostate is near the bladder, it could spread, what if it spread? They're going to have to take out my bladder. I'm going to be one of those old guys with a bag of urine on my leg. How the hell will that look at the beach? Oh my God, it's spread,* is the mantra I've got spinning around and around in my head. However, it didn't spread. I had the cystoscopy and it went off without a hitch (see previous chapter on what it's like to have a cystoscopy). Dr. Yalowitz is the kindest, warmest, sweetest man you'll ever meet. It's like your grandfather giving you a cystoscopy. Okay, I just threw up a little in my mouth. It's not like your grandfather giving you a cystoscopy. It's like a truly compassionate doctor who cares about your wellbeing giving you a cystoscopy. I feel blessed to have him on my side.

I have the cystoscopy, he wishes me well, tells me there is no cancer there, but I'm still in a funk. I know he's missed something. I'm in full-on negative mode as I pass the receptionist. Here's where a good doctor is not enough—a good office staff is an added plus. I stopped to say goodbye to the receptionist. She looked at me and asked how I was doing. I told her I was anxious and scared and falling into a deep depression. Her eyes filled up and she said, "You're going to be fine. I know this."

I thanked her and exited the office. As I'm walking to the elevator, the receptionist sticks her head out the office door and yells to me. I stop and turn. She walks up to me and puts her arms around me, "Mr. Bluestein. I'm gonna keep you in my prayers." She hugs me a little tighter, an act of kindness I will never forget. It comforted me to think that she would care enough to get up from her desk just to take care of my emotional needs. It made such an impact on me I almost cried. It comforted me. It gave me hope. I could never thank her enough. Karen, I love you.

Ok, cystoscopy on Friday, colonoscopy on Monday. It's my -oscopy weekend of fear and dread. I don't know if you ever have had a colonoscopy but I've had a few. Hey, you can't say I don't know how to have a good time. I know what to expect. Everyone says the same thing, "The procedure is nothing, it's the prep that sucks," and it does suck. Eight ounces of Gatorade every fifteen minutes. It's mixed with Miralax, which is sort of an intestinal power wash. You start nice and slow and then suddenly your stomach begins to rumble like Mount St. Helen and then there isn't a bathroom close enough. You expel things from your body that you haven't seen in years. I said to a friend, "I think I just saw pieces of my Bar Mitzvah cake." This routine goes on for hours until you are actually passing a clear liquid that looks like the East River in New York City. Your insides are so clean that on your X-ray there is now a sparkle emoji.

At six the next morning, I am up and waiting to go to the clinic where the colonoscopy will be done. A couple more runs to the bathroom, and I'm good to go. By the time I walk into the clinic it's 7 a.m. The place is packed with people who look like they're waiting to be questioned by the Spanish Inquisition. There's an empty void in their eyes because there's an empty void in their intestines because they've voided all night (see what I did there?).

I check in and wait to be called. Being a writer/comedian, I observe. I observe everything. The old man who left his hearing aids at home and is answering everything wrong, "When was the last time you ate?"

"Is it eight? Wow time really flies?"

I see the patients who had the 5 a.m. appointments coming out of recovery. They're walking with this shit-eating grin on their faces, you know, like it's the 1960s and they've just left Studio 54. The drugs they give you these days are truly wonderful. There's a silver lining to every dark cloud. I'll bet if I had these drugs in the 1960s, I'd be dead now. There's a nice thought going in. FYI—I can have medical drugs for this procedure and it doesn't interfere with my sobriety. See, I'm already finding the good in this experience. I'm about to get loaded on a free pass.

To get to the operating room there is a door that uses a push button code. I watch as nurse after nurse enters the code. Beep, beep, beep, beep… enter. Beep, beep, beep, beep… enter. Beep, beep, beep, beep… enter. Then this little short, fat guy tries to get in. He looks like one of the characters in a Mario Brothers video game: short, pot bellied, bald headed and dressed like Mario. He tries to get in. Beep, Beep, Beep…. "Bahhhh." Beep, Beep, Beep…. "Bahhhh." Beep, Beep, Beep…. "Bahhhh." Finally a nurse lets him in. I think to myself, *I wonder what does that moron does here? Probably a janitor.*

I am called to go in for my procedure. I meet Patricia, a gorgeous African American nurse who was warm, kind, and caring.

"Take off your clothes. Leave your socks on," she says like it's an episode of *Blackish*.

"I'm not wearing socks," I sheepishly reply.

"Oh, honey you're gonna be cold. It can get cold in here. Yep, man comes to surgery without socks. Hello!" She laughs and gives me a big hug, "Don't you worry, Baby man, I'll get you some booties."

She does, and I laugh at her personality as I strip down and climb into the bed. I'm left alone. Leaving me alone at this point is never a good thing. This is the worst time for me. This is when my mind goes to all kinds of bad places. It's my own personal hell as the committee between my ears goes into high gear. I'm lost in my negative thoughts when a fellow comes in (side note #1217, a fellow is a doctor. They have completed their internship and residency and want to gain more expertise in their specific field of medicine and so they work with and under another more established doctor). As luck would have it, this fellow was a woman—a woman who is a fellow—but this woman was so masculine she actually could have been a fellow. We exchange pleasantries and she leaves. Then the colonoscopy doctor sticks his head in.

"Hi, how ya doin'?" It's like they all want to meet the victim before the crime. He says some reassuring things like, "I haven't lost a patient yet." It's the "yet" that gets me. I think to myself, *There's always a first time.* He leaves and I'm left alone to think. I'm deep in thought about how I'm going to deal with my cancer and what it's going to do to my life and how it will change everything. Suddenly there is a calm in the room, and it makes me take notice. I feel a presence. Suddenly, I hear my Aunt Shirley's voice as clear as if she was standing in the room with me. "I'm right here with you, Stevie," she says in her warm reassuring voice. Aunt Shirley was my favorite aunt. She was the one who loved me the way I wanted to be loved as a child. When it was bad with my parents, I would always go to Aunt Shirley and she would always make it better. There was another reason I loved her so much—Aunt Shirley loved to laugh at my jokes. She encouraged me to follow my dream of a career in comedy. I burst into tears as these memories came pouring back to me. She had passed away four months prior to my colonoscopy and cancer diagnosis. As I'm crying like a baby, in walks one of the Mario Brothers. I think he's going to mop the floor. I recognized him immediately, he's the Beep, Beep, Beep…. "Bahhhh" guy. Oh my God! He's not a janitor. Oh my God! He's the anesthesiologist. *Oh my God!* The guy who can't get into the clinic because he can't figure out the code is going to put me under. *Michael Jackson, I'm coming!* He asks all the right questions and wants to know why I'm crying. I tell him about my fear of the cancer spreading and my aunt and how scared I am. "If there is something you could give me to calm me down I would really appreciate it," I say like a four year old asking for a cookie.

The doctor reaches into his pocket and pulls out a syringe. I'm thinking of the Carol Burnett sketch where Tim Conway is doing Harvey Corman's dental work and stabs himself with the needle. I laugh. I see this guy doing the same thing and falling asleep before he puts me to sleep. He doesn't ask why I'm laughing he just begins the injection.

The doctor puts the needle into my IV line. I turn to him and say, "Are you from New York, cause I lived in the city on East 58th Street....Zzzzzzzz." I'm out cold. The next thing I know, Shoshanna is waking me up and putting my clothes back on. That's the wonderful thing about modern medicine, when you have surgery you hear two things: "We're ready for you," and, "You can go home now." I don't remember going into the operating room, getting on the table, having the colonoscopy, going back to recovery. I remember nothing but the following words, "You were clear. No polyps. No cancer." A feeling of joy comes over me like I have not had in a long time. I hear Aunty Shirl say, "Told ya." I have passed the two most serious tests of my pre-prostate cancer surgery with flying colors. The cancer had not spread. I will now move on to the MRI and blood work with the worst behind me. Or so I thought.

The MRI From Hell

Despite the fact I have had a clear cystoscopy and colonoscopy, the doctors are covering all the bases. They want to see everything inside of me, so I am scheduled for an MRI. I don't know what they think they're going to find, maybe an Edible Arrangements franchise.

The instructions for the MRI are as follows: I am to make sure I do not eat after midnight. My appointment is at 6 p.m. the next day. That means I will not be able to eat all day. Let me tell you about my blood sugar—on a good day, my blood sugar drops like a stone off the Golden Gate Bridge. How the hell am I going to get through an entire day without eating and then add the time it takes to do the MRI? By the time they're done I'll be a limp dishrag. I decide to sleep the day away. You see, no energy burned, none needed to be replaced with a plate of pasta and French bread, a little cheese, maybe a cookie... see where I'm going here? At 5 p.m. I leave for the hospital; I see visions of cupcakes and half gallons of Byer's cookies and cream ice cream at every street corner. I see chicken wings and thighs, no wait those are pigeons. I'm so hungry I'm sucking on the dashboard of my friend's car—it's delicious by the way. Tastes like chicken. Why does everything taste like chicken? Ever have rabbit? Tastes like chicken? Shouldn't it taste like rabbit? When I cook I'm just happy that chicken tastes like chicken instead of inner tube.

In any case, I get to the hospital and I see the security guard. He's huge. I picture him with an apple in his mouth. I'm ready to eat the security guard—this guy could feed a family of nine for a month. I am told someone will contact me. Half an hour later I'm still waiting. I've started to get shaky and in a cold sweat. That's the first sign that the blood sugar is dropping. I go up to the receptionist and tell him that I have to be taken soon because my blood sugar is dropping fast. He makes a few phone calls and suddenly I'm being wheeled down a long corridor, a corridor I will never be able to find my way out of when the test is over. It's like I'm a test rat in a maze. If I make it back to the lobby, they'll give me pellets as a reward for finding my way home. Anyway, I'm taken to a room where there are lots of beds and as soon as I enter they are giving me crackers with peanut butter, an assortment of juices and puddings—lots and lots of pudding. I say, "The instructions told me I couldn't eat."

"Yeah, I don't know why they told you that. What favor ice cream do you want?"

What?? If I wasn't so weak I would have punched someone. Anger is also a sign of low blood sugar.

This Greek-looking guy comes over to tell me he will be the one to insert my IV. He really looked like a Greek God—very handsome—but when he opened his mouth, out came a Filipino cabin attendant on Crystal Cruise Line. I had to ask, "So, which one of your parents was from Greece?"

He looks at me. "How did you know?" Then I learn via a very long and very boring story of how his Greek father met his Filipino mother and how they fell in love and came to America and started a new life and had six children and were the best parents a boy could want. All I'm thinking is, *Just set up the fucking line, Apollo.* I have not had enough food, and I'm really, really grumpy. Duh!

Of the many tests that I must go through prior to surgery, the MRI is the most fun. They strap you to a board, put plugs in your ears, cover the plugs with head phones, and then begin giving you instructions, which are followed by you saying, "What? I can't hear you."

The test takes fourth-five minutes, in which your nose will begin to itch like it has never itched before in your life. Your arms are strapped to the table like you're about to have electric shock therapy and you are in a tube much like a birth canal. Suddenly the table is shaking—and I mean shaking like I thought we were having an earthquake. Yeah, that's where I want to be in an earthquake, strapped to a table in the basement of Cedars Sinai's Radiology Department. When they would finally find my body they'd say, "Here he is. He died of hunger." The table is shaking and this is after the technician telling me not to move or they will have to redo the test. You are shoved back and forth through this tube like a piston in a steam engine on the Titanic. It's boring. It's claustrophobic. It's cramped. It's like flying coach on American Airlines.

Then comes the contrast dye. "You're going to feel nauseous," says the Greek God.

"Oh really, because this has been so much fun so far," is what I want to say, but I don't want my sarcastic ass to be left in that tube strapped to a table as they go out to dinner. The tech doesn't tell you when they are injecting the dye. The machine does it automatically, you know, like a James Bond movie where the camera follows the liquid through the tube to the subject's heart until the subject is dead. Suddenly your arm is cold as the dye is let loose. I wait for the vomiting to begin. Nothing. I'm the one in a million who does not get sick from the dye. I guess it comes for decades of eating my mother's cooking. My mother was to cooking what The Rock is to Swan Lake.

The woman couldn't boil water and I'm sad to say I've inherited her skills in the kitchen. Winner!

The test is over in forty-five minutes. They pull me out of the birth canal. I expect one of them to hang me by my feet and slap me on the ass. Instead, they gently ask me to sit up. I do. I fall back down. I've had ice cream, cookies and cranberry juice. I'm lapsing into a sugar coma. They get me up and walk me around like it's the drunk tank at central jail, however, I'm fine and I'm ready to go home.

A male nurse takes me to the dressing room where he stands watching as I put on my underwear. In my head it's like the beginning of porn movie. Here's the scene, the male nurse stands watching, grinning, smirking, then suddenly a female nurse comes in. The two of them are watching, grinning smirking. There is a flash cut and suddenly the three of us are on the floor rolling around having wild passionate you-know. Back to reality. Jesus Christ if I don't eat something soon they are going to have to admit me to the hospital.

The male nurse then tells me how to get back to the lobby. I'm looking for the pellets again. They don't come. He says he'll walk me back so I can make it home safely, but first we stop at the feedback monitor where I am to rate my experience. I give them all tens. He's standing right there looking over my shoulder. What am I going to do, diss the whole experience? He could leave me there as punishment and I'd never find my way home.

Then he says, "There's one more category. Anyone you'd like to mention for outstanding service?" He smiles broadly.

"How do I spell your last name again?" I ask for the spelling of his last name like I've suddenly forgotten it. I never knew it. I haven't eaten. He types his name in. I think this is a good way to judge how the hospital is doing. Not. This is like the Lexus survey you get three days after you get your car. The dealer tells you the survey is coming and he tells you what the best answers should be. This survey is so biased they should just let the dealership fill it out themselves, which they sometimes actually ask permission to do.

I complete the hospital survey and the nurse escorts me back to the Lobby. I have completed one more test before my surgery on October 27th. The journey continues.

Waiting for GODOT

Everything is done. The pre-op tests are done. The post-op Jell-O has been purchased and stocked at my house like we're expecting a hurricane. The kitchen looks like the recovery room kitchen at the Camden Surgery Center in Beverly Hills where the stars get their faces lifted. There are more soft foods in that fridge than at assisted living in Boca Raton. Everything is done; all I have to do now is wait. That is the most difficult part of this whole journey. The waiting. Waiting for Friday, waiting to be checked in, waiting for the first IV, waiting for the night in the hospital where I am sure I'll contract the flesh-eating virus. Waiting. Just waiting has me in such a depression I can't function.

I was supposed to go to a Prostate Support Group the night before the surgery. Doesn't Prostate Support Group sound like a room full of jock straps sitting around talking about their latest prostate problem? It's not, it's a group of men who get together to discuss their leaking, their diapers, and a life without hard-ons. Fun group. I guess the People Without Arms and Legs support group was out on their bowling night. I was supposed to go to the prostate group the night before surgery but I couldn't get myself out of the chair. I was so depressed I couldn't move. I sat in that chair in the living room reviewing my life, thinking about the people I've lost, wanting my mother

29

to be there knowing all the time that even if she was there she would not be able to console me because she just didn't have that kind of warmth for me in her DNA. I called the leader of the group to tell him I wasn't coming and expecting to get some comforting words of wisdom on my condition, something to make me feel better the night before surgery. This is what I got, "I know how you're feeling, when I was at that stage all I could think of was they're going to rip my prostate out of my body. And the pain and discomfort I'm going to experience afterwards is going to be hell. Who wants to go through that? And why did this have to happen to me?" This was from the support group president. Who needs support like that? If I wanted support like that, I'd call my family.

Earlier in the day, as I sat at my desk trying to focus and pay some bills. I heard "Stephen, it's your Mutha," and I heard it as clear as a bell (she had a thick Boston accent). She offered no words of consolation. She couldn't do that when she was alive, she certainly can't do it now that she's dead. She was letting me know that she was around and watching over me. For those who don't believe in such crap, skip to the next paragraph. I didn't believe in it either. To me, death was final, and it is until you start getting those messages they give you. Oh yes, they give messages and they are as clear as a bell. You'll know them when they happen because it is so personal. Like in this case, one word from my mutha and I slumped into a deeper depression and was not able to pull myself out of it. No matter what I did or how hard I tried, I was depressed. She was the cause. She was here. I knew it. That was her message. I would have preferred a dove landing on my coffee table, but that's not what our relationship was about. I am just one of those people who grew up nurture-starved. I think it is why I ended up on stage. All that love coming back over the footlights was what I needed so desperately. I have learned a big lesson in my many years—the depression will pass. It will pass and I will come through this surgery being better on the other side. Yeah, right. I just cannot shake this feeling of impending doom. It hangs over me like a dark cloud filled with fear and anxiety and loneliness. No matter how many friends call to tell me they love me, no matter how many batches of cookies are delivered, no matter how many (in the hundreds) of well wishes I am getting, I cannot feel any of it on this day before surgery. Why would I? I never learned what nurturing is. I don't know how to accept it or what to do with it, so I simply move forward the best that I can. I move forward and get to the day of surgery one day at a time. What else can I do?

More on the Depression Because the Last Chapter Wasn't Depressing Enough

I have battled depression all of my life. Depression and anxiety were my make-believe friends as a child. They were always there with me. With incredible therapy, I have learned how to handle them. When I say incredible therapy, let me just say there are whole wings of psychiatrist's homes that were financed on the back of my childhood, "Come in, we call this the Bluestein wing." So I know depression; but I have never ever had a depression like the one I experienced the night before the surgery.

I was having the kind of depression where the simplest mention of a name or a date sends me running to the bathroom for tissues. Early in the day I got a haircut and cried at the barbershop because I saw my first grey hair. The night before, at 4 a.m., I woke up from a sound sleep crying. What was I crying about? Oh I don't know, maybe I was upset about missing that field trip to Cape Cod in the sixth grade because I had the measles. Trust me, it was important.

I am trying to put a finger on why I was feeling so low. Was it the realization that I actually am growing older? Was it the loss of the use of my penis (not that it's been so busy of late, but still, it's nice to have one when you need it…. Guys, back me up here)? I just don't know what it was. The best theory I have is that I don't feel there is anyone who truly cares about me. Now, if that's not the most insane thing I've ever written, I don't know what is. The outpouring of love was incredible. Every day phone calls and cards came into the house. Every day I got private messages on Facebook. Every day packages arrive—and every day I feel as empty as Trump's empathy sack.

How does one get that way? Does it really matter? What matters is what I do to fight the depression. Why the depression is here is really of no consequence. Dealing with it is. Sharing helps. I will share with anyone. At Ralphs Grocery Store the checker said, "Do you have any coupons?"

To which I replied, "No but I have a Groupon for 50% off cancer."

She looked at me like I was insane, which, of course, I am, but it did put a smile on her face and that's what I'm all about, making you laugh. That's what makes me happy, making you happy.

When my doctor heard about my depression he immediately ordered some anti-depressants for me. I cancelled the order. Why? I have friends on anti-depressants, and they're some of the most insane people I know. They are crazy when they're not on drugs, and they are even crazier on the anti-depressants. I don't know a single person who took an anti-depressant, settled down, and won the Noble Peace Prize for being normal. Mostly what happens is they take the anti-depressant and call me at three in the morning to tell me they are going to kill themselves. When I tell them I'll be right over they happily say, "That's not necessary. I'm better now." Only now I can't sleep cause it's four a.m. and the dog is circling the bed thinking it's time to get up and he wants to be fed... or else.

I said to a friend, "Did you ever feel like your life was dragging along like you were on hold for Spectrum technical support?" The waiting is a nightmare. Each day I learned something that I hadn't learned before about my surgery. For instance, I was told today that my testicles will swell up like basketballs. I don't know if you know this about me, but I'm not into sports. What the hell am I going to do with two basketballs? The paperwork says, "Rest them on a towel." Sure, but how's that going to look at Bloomingdales?

I cannot tell you how much I wanted this over and done with. Once it's done and there is no turning back I will be okay. Once it's done and I have no alternative but to start my new life and deal with what life has given me, I'll be okay. Once I take the noose down from over the rafter, the world will look like a brighter place.

That's what I was dealing with the day before surgery—depression, anxiety, sadness. Can't live with them, can't live without them, but I'd be willing to try.

The Day of the Surgery or How I Lost My Prostate In the Parking Lot of Cedars

Nothing to eat after midnight! That's what it says on the pre-surgery slip. Nothing to eat or drink after midnight! What is it with these doctors? I can't eat after midnight? They're out having dinner with their friends. I'm on the floor of my bedroom because I don't have the strength to get up to wash my face, because I can't eat after midnight. So what did I do? I eat right up to 11:59 p.m. I stuffed more crap into my stomach than it's seen in decades. I go to sleep and I am up at 7:00 a.m. starving. I have never been this hungry in my life. Me, who usually eats maybe a single piece of toast for breakfast, wakes up this morning wanting a truck driver's diner breakfast from Denny's, and I can't eat, and the surgery isn't until 2:00 p.m. At this point I'll do anything to subdue my hunger. I'm sucking on pieces of furniture. I try napping. I'm sucking on the pillow. It doesn't work, I dream about eating. I wake up with a pillowcase in my mouth. It's my own personal pre-surgery hell.

I'm watching the clock like I'm on death row. How could it possibly be only five minutes later than it was before? I need to eat something. I check the paperwork again. I can take a sip of water with my pills. I already took my pills. What constitutes a sip? How much is a sip? What's the difference between a sip and a slurp? Now I'm pacing around the house trying to keep my mind off the surgery. I've organized my office. I've vacuumed the back yard. That's right, I dragged the upright vacuum out into the middle of the patio and vacuumed the patio. Even the dogs are embarrassed at these insane actions.

Finally it's 1:00 p.m. and I can leave for the hospital. A dear friend is driving me. He carries my suitcase with the overnight essentials. We enter the front door of Cedars where a sweet elderly man asks me what he can do for me. I answer, "Cancel my surgery." He doesn't react. I guess he's heard this joke before. I give him my name. He types in BLOOMSTEEN. I correct him. He types in, BLUEMSTEEN. I finally show him my driver's license. He says, "What an odd way to spell that." Shoot me. Just fucking shoot me now.

He finds my chart and tells me I will be escorted up to the admitting office by one of their volunteers. An elderly Spanish man takes us up to the office and tells me to "Esit. Esomeone will be right wit ju." Within ten minutes my name is called and I am escorted into a private office where I am asked to show my photo I.D. Like someone is going to sneak in and try to steal my prostate surgery. Who would try to have their prostate taken out instead of me? Who steals prostate surgery? What has this world come to when a hospital has to make sure someone isn't trying to rip off your prostate surgery? The nurses are upstairs stuffing their purses with Keri Lotion but this woman is worried someone is coming to take my place. It's absolutely insane.

The intake takes only a few minutes and we are escorted to the waiting room to the pre-op surgical suite. A Filipino male nurse comes out to greet me. He is wearing more make up than Ru Paul. It's subtle but in the right light of day you can see the line under his chin where the make up stops and the five o'clock shadow begins. I start looking for the hidden cameras. Maybe I don't have prostate cancer. Maybe they are doing all this so I can be a mark on *Punk'd*. No, it's for real. I am being taken to the pre-op room by a drag queen who didn't have enough time to get home and take off his makeup after lip syncing Bette Midler at his show last night.

The nurse gives me my instructions and leaves me alone in the room. It's there I remember what I forgot to do at the house. In the rush to get to the hospital I had forgotten to drop to my knees and ask God for his will in my life. From the day I got sober it's something I do when life is too much for me. I knew I had to find a quiet place where I could be alone and have my time with my God. The nurse came back and asked if I had to go to the bathroom before the surgery. Bingo! I had my private time. I went into that surgical bathroom with its yellow tile floors and anti-bacterial hand sanitizer and I dropped to my knees. I told God I would accept his will in my life and I was ready to take this challenge one day at a time. It only took three minutes for me to connect with a higher power, but I did. When the nurse knocked on the door I knew that I was ready to face whatever was ahead of me. Just to make the bathroom trip look real, I flushed the toilet and exited the bathroom wiping my hands. I'm so detailed oriented when I'm making up a lie.

I am escorted back to my bed. Once you are in the pre-op area they never leave you alone. It's like they fear you're going to flee for your life and screw up their operating schedule. I am escorted back to my bed and forced to strip naked and put on a gown. Why they call it a gown is beyond me. Cinderella ain't wearing this to the ball. "Who's the beautiful young girl with her ass exposed?" asks the Prince. I lie in the bed and suddenly there are all kinds of technicians around me poking, sticking, hooking me up to machines. It's at this point I no longer feel like a person but more like a slab of meat they are working on to wash and prepare for cooking. I guess they've done this so many times the patient ceases to be human and more like a thing. Lying in that bed I have never felt more human in my life, or more vulnerable. I'm wearing one of those caps the cafeteria ladies wear. My anxiety level is a 12.9 on a scale of one to ten. I want to jump out of the bed and run down the hall like in one of those madcap comedies we all hate to love. I wanted to flee the hospital and pretend I didn't have cancer. I wanted to be anywhere but where I was at that very moment. But the reality was I did have cancer and there was nowhere to go but on a gurney and into the operating room.

As my mind was racing a mile a minute this saint of a woman comes up to my bedside. She must have been in her early thirties with the face of an angel. Her dark brown hair framed her gorgeous brown eyes. Her fair skin seemed like silk as she took my hand. Her voice was soothing. Her bedside manner was gentle and reassuring. It was just what I needed at that very moment.

"Let me guess... you're the fellow," I guess.

She smiles and sheepishly says, "No, I'm the anesthesiologist."

I fear that I've just insulted her but she is so sweet and so kind that she gives me no indication that has happened. I add, "I only said fellow because the fellow is always the first doctor to come and visit before the surgery."

She smiles but I know she hates me despite her warm smile and that she'll accidentally overdose me in surgery. The one person you don't want to piss off is the anesthesiologist. She asks how I'm doing and I tell her that my anxiety level is off the charts and that I'm scared to death and that I don't want to be there and why did this have to happen to me and where are the drugs that colonoscopy doctor gave me? Where are they, God damnit! She warmly smiles at me like she's known me all my life and takes my hand. "I will not let anything happen to you."

When she says it I know she means it, my overdose fears are gone. I begin to calm down. We chat some more and I learn she is Armenian. Since my closest and dearest friends for the last thirty-five years are Armenian, we make an immediate connection. I feel myself relaxing even more and it has nothing to do with the drugs she had just injected into my IV line. I see this calmness as one of those signs I am always looking for. My Aunt Shirley has brought me an angel of an Armenian to guide me through the surgery. I have found my sign and it was all I needed to relax. The last thing I remember is this wonderful woman looking at me and smiling. I remember nothing else from the moment on. The drugs had kicked in. When I say I remember nothing, I mean nothing. Don't remember seeing the doctor prior to surgery. Don't remember being wheeled into the O.R. It's like the whole experience has been cleared from my brain so I can't relive it or so that it no longer can cause me anxiety. That's the miracles of modern medicine!

After the Surgery. Get the Number of That Truck

The next thing I know I'm in a hospital room. It's a private room, small but ample and it's on the eighth floor at Cedars. The eighth floor of Cedars is like The Ritz Carlton of hospital floors. It's the floor where the food is a little better and the nurses are a little more attentive. Fuck it, I'll just say it. It's the celebrity floor. The institutional walls are painted a soothing cream color. They don't want you coming out of surgery and looking at magenta walls. The TV hangs from the ceiling like they always do only it's a little better TV than the other floors. I have a view from my window of—get ready for it—the other wing of the hospital. There are patients looking at me as I'm looking at them. It's like we are a fraternity of sick people looking at each other for some way to escape, and waving, "Hiiiii! How's your surgery?"

I have a bladder bag and much to my surprise the room is filled with friends. I am told that I have been telling everyone in the recovery room that I loved them all. I have no memory of this but it makes me happy that I was so grateful for the care I was getting and letting them know. It could have been much more ugly. It could have been, "Your mother sucks cocks in hell," but it wasn't, and I am happy I was on my best behavior. Truth be told, I was so happy that I was alive after the surgery that I *did* love them all. I was glad that I thanked them for getting me through this major event in my life. It wasn't drugs at all that was making me say I love you. I was actually being grateful for their care.

The first thing I do remember was that I felt no pain. I was expecting to be in major pain after surgery but I had none. Little did I know that I had been pumped up with more painkillers than it took to take down King Kong. I was flying like a kite. They do that now so that after surgery you are not in too much discomfort. I was very happy they developed that protocol because I'm not good with pain. You know how in the movies Bruce Willis tries to stop the terrorist and they shoot him up but he keeps on going? Ya, I'm not like that. I have an ingrown toenail and I'm in a wheelchair whining, so I was wildly happy that I was in no pain at all.

The friends stay a bit longer and then the nurse tells them I need to rest and one by one they leave me so I can get some sleep. Suddenly I am left alone in a room where a nurse comes in every fifteen minutes to make sure I'm okay—to change my IV bag or to wake me to give me a sleeping pill. Why do they do that? I had always heard about that happening and I thought it was a joke, but no, it's real. They come in to wake you to give you a sleeping pill. It's not a joke.

Next morning the food comes. Two pancakes that were so hard the *Our Gang* kids used them as wheels on their go-cart. I could not get them down. They stuck somewhere in my throat and just lodged there until I could wash them down with water. I suppose I could talk about hospital food but why discuss something that has been discussed for decades. Listen, you don't go into the hospital because of the cuisine, and if you do, you don't need Cedars, you need a padded room in a psychiatric ward. The food was inedible. It looked like food, it smelled like food, it didn't taste like food. I don't know if it was the medication or the fact that opening my eyes took every ounce of strength I had, but I could not get that food down. I grew weak because of it. Add to that, my mouth was so dry I could barely swallow, and they want me to eat lasagna like it's the Feast of San Gennaro. Well they called it lasagna but it tasted like the inside of a Humvee wheel well. Who do they have cooking in that kitchen, trained apes? Friends snuck in real food—food with texture and taste and color—something the cooks at the hospital had never seen before. I took a picture and sent it to them. If it weren't for my wonderful compadres I would have died of starvation in that hospital and with no prostate. I thought to myself, *And this is the eighth floor where the food is supposed to be the best in the hospital. Can you imagine what they're getting on the second floor... gruel?* In my mind I see patients sitting on the corridor floor begging for food, "Alms... alms for the poor. Can you spare a biscuit?"

Despite the food, I was doing fine until the male nurse came in to tell me, "You need to walk."

"You walk. I'm fine here in bed," is what I wanted to say, but, "Okay," is all I could get out. Why am I such a people pleaser? I didn't want to walk. I didn't want to move, but there I was getting out of that bed less than twenty-four hours after surgery. I'm supposed to walk the entire eighth floor with its fancy rooms and walls of expensive art. I looked down at the end of the hall—it was so far away it ended in a vanishing point. Then I learn that when we get to the end of that hallway we will turn right and walk the next hall until I walk the entire length of the eighth floor. There is no way I am going to do this, but I don't let the nurse know. Fuck him. He'll learn soon enough.

There I am with my walker, walking down the hallway at Cedar's. Ninety year-old women are passing me in their wheel chairs screaming, "Out of my way, slow boy!" I am hit with a big dose of reality. My eyes begin to well up as I see my grandfather in front of me. He's walking down a hall with a walker and then I realized it's a mirror. It's me walking down that corridor. I am now my grandfather. As I see the image, I feel so alone. I want someone there who really loves me and is rooting me for me. I want them to be on this first walk with me but all I had was the male nurse who was as kind as he could be to a stranger. I am also reminded that the male nurse would have been kinder to me than my parents who had the nurturing skills of a pit bull, "Come on, they only took out your prostate...what's the big deal?"

We make it three quarters of the way up that first hallway and I say, "I'm done." I was having a lot of pain where the catheter entered my body. He doesn't fight me and we turn back to my room where I climb into bed like I've just climbed Mount Everest without the assistance of a Sherpa. He tells me that I was having pain because the tip of my schvantz needed to be lubricated. I look at him and say, "Not without dinner and a movie first."

The nurse starts to laugh and continues to laugh as the other nurse comes into the room, "You two are having too much fun."

To which I say, "And the fun is just about to begin... go get the lube."

Now they are both laughing. See, I live to make you laugh, even if I'm in pain. As they are working their magic on the lubrication the female nurse says, "It's a wonderful thing to have a sense of humor when you've just come out of surgery." I explain that it's just how I'm hard wired. I see things and my mind finds the funny in it. I was once having some dental work done where I needed to be put out. As the anesthesia was wearing off I turned to the dentist and said, "While you were in there, you didn't happen to find my garage opener did you?" He laughed and told me in thirty-five years of dental surgery he had never had a patient come out of anesthesia and crack a joke. That's just me. My mind works differently than most people. While my mother found it embarrassing and never once encouraged me, it's what fueled my career and got me that big house in Bel Air and the Tesla. So there!

I was supposed to go home the next day but the "numbers" were off. What does that mean, "The numbers are off?" Who is taking care of me, a Bookie? I was assured it was because of the anesthesia but they wanted to keep me another day until every thing was perfect. They kept me that extra day, a day in which I was used as a human pincushion. Don't you love it when the nurse says, "Wow your veins have really collapsed. This is going to be tough," and then goes digging for a vein like she's at the beach looking for clams? Two days after I got home my arm was black and blue from the wrist to the elbow. I digress. I was a prince of a patient. I didn't complain. I didn't cry. I just let them do what they were supposed to do. After all, when I said my prayer in the pre-op bathroom I did say, "Your will in my life," and so if this what was supposed to happen I couldn't complain, and I didn't.

I want to go on record right here and now. The nursing staff at Cedars are some of the finest professionals I have ever had the pleasure of meeting. I am not easy to please and these nurses, to a person, were warm and caring and supportive and loving. They let you know they were there to make you feel better and that nothing was too much to ask from them. I don't think I could have made it that first couple of nights in the hospital if it wasn't for that wonderful army of nurses who took care of me like I was a long-lost relative.

A little later in the day the doctors come in to check on me. At one point three doctors came in and I dubbed them the cast of *E.R.* I have never seen three more gorgeous people in my life. I thought they were going to give me their 8x10s instead of a check-up. There were two male doctors and one female. She was auburn-haired and quite beautiful. The male doctors were also quite handsome, a Korean man who looked like the guy from *LOST* and Middle-Eastern looking guy who will have his own TV series within five years. Hey, it's Hollywood, everyone wants to be in show business. I joked with them because that's what I do. I asked if they had come from central casting. The two men laughed. The woman did not, she was all business. She would have none of this class-clowning I was so well known for. "I am doctor..." and she gave me her name as she extended her hand like we were meeting to close a real estate deal. "We see you are progressing well... you should be out of here soon." No smile. No warmth; all business. They asked if I had any questions.

"Yes, why do I feel this bad?"

"Mr. Bluestein, you just had major surgery," she said. Major Surgery? Those two words were never spoken when I first met with the surgeon three weeks prior. Maybe if I had heard "major surgery" I would have given this whole experience a second thought, but what am I musing about that now for? My prostate is in a jar somewhere at Cedars. Deal with what you have been given, Steve. I smiled and nodded. They stayed a few minutes and then left as quickly as they came. It was like, who were those masked people? And get the name of that truck.

I stayed in the hospital for two days. On the second day the Korean doctor came in wearing golf clothes. Why are all the doctors in golf clothes? Is that a class in medical school? "Golf and the patient release." He told me the numbers were back to normal and I could go home. I can't tell you how happy I was. Home. When I think of home I think of a place with central vacuuming and enough dog hair to weave a comforter (Interesting side note #11: I have a golden retriever—the most wonderful dog on the planet—who sheds hair by the bucket-full on a daily basis. I think they should change the name of that dog to the golden shedder). The paper work was signed, the bags were packed, a nurse was there to take me to my car. I climbed into that wheelchair with all the gusto of road kill. I don't remember the ride down from the room to the car. I don't remember going through the lobby or getting into my car. My room was on the eighth floor so I know they didn't lower me down to the street on a rope. I must have taken the elevator but I remember nothing. All I remember is that Sunset Blvd. needs to be repaved because I felt every bump in that road on the ride home.

Upon arrival to my home, I suddenly became aware of the sixteen steps that I would have to climb to get into my house. I was determined to get into my own bed and so I made the climb with every ounce of strength I had left. Let me describe the assent. Step. Scream. Step. Scream. Step. Scream. Sixteen times.

At the first landing, and for the first time in my life, I felt myself falling backward with no control of my body. It's like I wasn't there to control my limbs. Thank God a friend was there to pull me forward by grabbing my shirt. I took a minute on the landing to understand what had just happened. I had almost fallen backwards down the first eight steps. This was way more serious than I thought it was going to be. For the first time "major surgery" sank in.

We progressed up the second flight of stairs and I made it into my bed. I won't lie, I cried like a baby when I got home. I don't know if it was the relief of having the surgery behind me or the gratitude I felt for all the love that had been thrown my way or if I was simply spent and my emotions were finally coming to the surface. Whatever it was, I was glad to be home and in my own bed. I was anxious to see my dogs and so I called for them, the Golden Retriever came running along with his best pal the Bichon. As soon as they heard my voice my dogs were at my side. On a regular day they would jump on the bed and lie on my chest or on my legs but dogs know when something is wrong with their master. They ran into the bedroom and suddenly stopped like they had been commanded to do so. Then Louie, the Bichon, jumped up on the bed and slowly approached me. On any given day that dog would have bolted to me and climbed up on my chest so he could snuggle his head into my neck, but today he slowly approached me, smelled around the blanket and then looked me right in the eyes. Without me saying anything he gently laid down beside me. That dog stayed off my chest and tender areas for almost two weeks. On the day that I got out of bed and went into the living room to sit in a big cushy chair, he followed me, jumped up on the arm of the oversized chair and gently put a paw on my stomach. When I told him it was okay, that I didn't hurt anymore, he moved from the arm of the chair into my lap where he curled into a ball and stayed there until I was ready to move again. The other dog, who is over seventy-five pounds, stayed by my side the entire time I was in bed. He never moved away from me. Even when it was time to eat his dinner he would come over to me, put his head on my hand as if to say, "I'm going now but I'll be right back." Then he left to have his dinner only to return to his spot on the side of the bed where he could guard me until I was able to take care of myself again. It was the kind of love that only a dog can give, and that's the reason I have been a dog owner for over forty years. I was never more grateful to have the two I have now than those first two weeks home after surgery. It centered me. They gave me companionship. They gave me love. I was incredibly grateful.

What I was not grateful for was the fricken bladder bag—or the

Foley catheter as it is named. Dr. Frederick Foley invented it in 1929. That's his claim to fame along with a few other medical inventions, but it was his bag full of piss that he will forever be remembered for, especially by yours truly. I wonder how his kids felt.

"What does your dad do?"

"Oh my dad? He...uh... he invents things."

"What kid of things?"

"Oh just things. Medical things."

"Why are you being so evasive? What does your Dad invent?"

"Fine! He invented a thing that goes into your bladder and collects your urine."

Silence.

"Your father was Frederick Foley?"

"Yeah. Wanna do something about it?"

End scene.

Unless you've been hooked up to a Foley bag via your genitals you don't know what hell is. It has to be emptied. It has to be carried. It has to be disguised when people come to visit because it makes them vomit. It's a constant reminder that you had major surgery and that back to normal was not just around the corner, it was *way* down the road. I hated that bag. I hated Dr. Foley. I hated the whole experience. I hated being tied down to a bag of urine and what it represented, but there was nothing I could do about it. It was there and I had to deal with it and I did deal with it to the best of my ability.

When the doctor first told me about the Foley he said, "It's not that bad. We'll give you one that straps to your leg and you'll be able to go out in public and no one will know you have it on."

I said, "Right! And I'll be at the mall and the bag will burst and I'll be standing there screaming, 'Bad dog! Bad dog!'"

Nothing. No laugh. Why do I even try with this guy?

I had friends stay with me in the house. You never know who loves you until you've seen your homeboy don rubber gloves and pour the contents of your urine bag into a basin. I am truly blessed to have friends that are closer than family. Now back to my prostate saga.

That first night home I thought I was going to die. I couldn't sleep in my bed because of the Foley. It was always in the way and when I tried to roll onto my side it was like someone was shoving a red-hot poker into my groin. Well not really groin—I'm being polite here. That first night I slept seated in an armchair in the living room with two pillows behind me and my feet up on an ottoman with the bladder bag hanging off the knob of the custom-made barrel table my Aunt Shirley had ordered for her first home on Long Island that I later inherited as she upgraded from one home to another and donated her furniture to my mother, and I got it when my mother died. How's that for a run-on sentence?

Sleeping in an armchair doesn't seem like it should be comfortable, but it was. I would doze off and open my eyes and look over into the kitchen where my friend James would be sitting. That man sat up until almost five in the morning just watching over me. I finally said to him, "Go to sleep. I'm fine," and he reluctantly went up to the guest bedroom to catch up on the sleep he had lost. Never in my life had I had that kind of care. It was the kind of friendship I wish for all of you. The kind where just knowing your friend is around makes you feel warm inside…. Or was that the pee?

Strangely enough, I was actually able to get a full night's sleep. I guess it was that and the anesthesia that was still in my system along with a blood pressure of 115/55. I have battled high blood pressure for decades and suddenly had the blood pressure of a corpse. My body was doing all kinds of strange and miraculous things—none of which I wanted it to do. I just wanted to feel better. I am very impatient, but with this surgery there could be no impatience. I could not rush this thing. I had to let time heal. Oh wait. I guess that's where that expression comes from—time heals all wounds. See? I'm learning something new every day.

The First Week... Should Be
the First Weak

The first week was a series of highs and lows. The lows started as the anesthesia left my body. Suddenly the miracle of painlessness abandoned me and hello, agony came to visit. I was taking pain pills with such regularity you could set your watch. I actually did set my watch to chime when it was time to take another pill. The problem with the pills was, they make you constipated, so along with the pain pills I was taking stool softener. Don't you wish they actually had stool softeners for bar stools? Those damn things are so uncomfortable to sit on while hitting on the drunk sitting next to you. The stool softeners were followed by a laxative. You combine a stool softener and a laxative and one good fart could blow the windows out in your bedroom. So it was painkillers, laxatives, and stool softeners along with my regular blood pressure pills and statins for cholesterol. When I compare the drugs I took in the 1960s to the drugs I'm taking now, I want to cry. Talk about the circle of life! I had come full circle from the recreational drugs of the 1960s to the stuff you see advertised in AARP magazines.

Let me tell you about the highs. When you are sick and in pain, when you are feeling so low and alone that you know no one cares, and then the doorbell rings and it's a delivery person with a platter of some incredible food thing—is there nothing more wonderful?? Now let me tell you about these deliveries. First came the cookies, they were delivered in something that looked like a float from the Rose Bowl Parade. It was huge and had every kind of cookie you could think of: chocolate chip, macadamia nut, chocolate-chocolate chip, oatmeal raisin. They weren't those skimpy little one-bite cookies either, they were the kind you had to hold in both hands and wash down with two glasses of milk. These were big ones—cookies that could put a diabetic into a coma. The platter was so big that for exercise I would walk around it just to get in a little cardio.

More important than the cookies or how big they were, was the fact that they were a constant reminder that someone really cared. It was a reminder that when you really need your friends, they are there for you. These reminders continued every day for the next couple of weeks because the next few day, a platter of muffins the size of Rhode Island was delivered. I was in shock, sugar shock. I had just had six cookies. The ocean of love didn't stop there. The day after that, a huge chocolate cake was delivered to my front door. Huge! It was the kind of cake they use after the opening night of a Broadway show. It was cake for 400 people and all I had was myself, a glass of milk, and really big fork. I was high with joy—but the kind of high you won't get arrested for while driving. That high happened over and over again— food, balloons, cakes, candy, deli, flowers—the stream of well wishes was non-stop. I called each of these wonderful friends who made sure I knew I was loved and told them how much their efforts meant to me. On each call I cried like a baby. One friend even said to me, "This isn't like you," and it wasn't, I don't cry. I make others cry. For the first time in my life I was so overwhelmed with gratitude that my emotions were on the surface and showed themselves with tears of joy.

On the Internet, Facebook exploded with well-wishes and love. It was embarrassing, because before I went into the hospital I sent out a letter to my closest friends and then posted the letter on Facebook. It went something like, "Ya know how some people like to be left alone when they are sick? I am not one of those people! I want flowers, I want cards, I want one of those things that looks like flowers but is actually cantaloupe." It got a huge laugh from all who read it. You see, I had asked for love because I never thought anyone would care about me. I truthfully never expected to get anything in return. When the tidal wave of love came flooding back over me, I was blown away with wonder and awe. You should have seen how many cantaloupes I had. It was hysterical. It was the yin to the yang of the pain and discomfort I was experiencing from the surgery. If each of us only knew how a little act of kindness can lift the spirit of a sick person, or how a phone call can let someone know that you're thinking about them and make them happy, or how a note saying, "Thinking of you," can bring a smile to the face of someone in need, then maybe many of us would do it more often. Kindness. It's the best thing you can give someone when they are ill, and I had kindness by the boatload. By the way, a little advice to anyone about to have prostate surgery—the letter really worked. I'm going to use it again if I ever have my gallbladder out.

I want to make sure you know how serious I am about the care I got from others. I joke about the cantaloupe, but it truly was the most healing experience. When you have felt so alone your entire life, when you're in your room and wondering if anyone cares, when the darkness fills your heart, these little acts of kindness become mountains of kindness. They can take a sad situation and turn it into a birthday party of joy and happiness. I have thanked those that were so kind to me. I have told them what their acts of kindness did for me. I hope they get the depth of emotion that comes with that thank-you because if it were not for my friends in that first week after surgery, I don't think I would have made it. As for my family, well they know exactly what they did. Nothing. I'm not bitter. It's just a lesson learned and put in a place where it will not be forgotten.

That's how the first week went: gratitude, sleeping in a chair, gratitude, pills, and pain (Interesting side note #236: The good thing about pain is that you can't remember it after it's gone. So when it's done you never have to experience it again. That's a little bit of information you might be able to use some day. You're welcome). I waited for the day when the pain would be gone. I waited every day, all day, for a week. I waited for that time when I could not remember the pain again. I thought it would never come, but eventually it came. I woke up one morning and thought, *I'm feeling better*. The sun was shining. The birds were singing. I sat up in bed and thought, *Thank you, God. I'm gonna make it through this with a little help from my friends*. There were so many friends who were there for me. Ben Blake was a general during my recuperation. He drove me to every doctor's appointment. He helped me up stairs. He was there every step of the way. I just needed to make sure he knew how much that constant support meant to me.

Week Two. Now What We Do?

I have been in bed for a week now. Things are going as they should go. I know I have a post-op appointment in the second week but no one has called to confirm, and quite frankly, I was too debilitated to do any follow-up. Then out of the blue I get a phone call from the doctor's office, "Mr. Bluestein, the doctor would like you to have some blood work done before you come in for your two week appointment. Can you go over to the Cedars lab and have the blood drawn before your next appointment?"

Long pause. I am trying to process what I am hearing. They want me to get out of bed and go to Cedars, walk from the parking structure to the lab, go up in an elevator while carrying my Foley bag, and give blood? As calmly as I can, I reply, "Are you out of your mind? I can't walk from my bed to the kitchen, which is about seventy feet, and you want me to go to Cedars fifth floor and have blood drawn? There is no way I can do that! I don't think you understand how weak I am. Can't a nurse come to the house?"

Long pause, "No. We don't do that," and it's said with the, "No. We don't do that, you moron." Understood.

We are at an impasse because I can't deal with this kind of ignorance. I tell her as politely as I can that I will get back to her. I was fuming. It wasn't so much that she didn't understand, it was her tone of voice, her "I don't care" attitude. I had just been through the worst week of my life and she was treating it like I got a bad haircut. I was distraught. I didn't know what to do. How could I possibly make the walk to the lab? The lab? How could I make the walk from the parking structure to the building? From the parking structure to the building, are you kidding me, I need Uber to get from the bedroom to the bathroom and I have an en suite at my house.

God has put some truly wonderful people in my life. Sue Kogen is another one of those people. Sue is married to Arnie Kogen, who is a three-time Emmy winning writer, and Sue is one of the top real estate brokers in Los Angeles. She's also like the mother I never had. I adore her. So, I called Sue Kogen. I knew if there was anyone who could have a solution for this problem, it's Sue Kogen. I tell her my dilemma and without batting an eye she says, "Call Cedars, tell them what you need, and they will set up a Medicare home healthcare nurse to your house."

"They will?" I ask like some first grader learning the alphabet.

"Yes, they will." She purrs. You see, a mom always has the solution, and Sue is one of the best.

I called Cedars, and sure enough they set up a home healthcare nurse for me without asking questions and with no problems at all. Within twenty-four hours a home healthcare nurse was in my house taking the blood needed for the appointment. When I tell you she was a dream-come-true, I would not be fibbing. A sweeter, more loving person I have never met. I could not have made it through that second week if she had not come to my house to not only draw blood, but to get me out of bed and walk me around the house. As the phrase goes, she was just what the doctor ordered. I am forever grateful to that wonderful lady for all she did for me through my recovery.

I was not looking forward to that second week appointment for many reasons. Forget the mean nurse I would have to deal with at the doctor's office, this was the week the Foley catheter came out. Don't get me wrong, I wanted it to come out, but I wasn't looking forward to the pain that it would cause me when it finally was removed. Let me just say, there are people on death row who are looking forward to their last meal with more gusto. I had heard all kinds of horror stories. I asked friends who had the surgery and had the Foley removed, "So what's it like? Does it hurt?"

To a person they said the same thing, "Take a pain pill before you see the doctor."

So that's exactly what I did. I went to have my catheter removed two sheets to the wind. That doctor could have removed my arm from the socket and I wouldn't have felt it. Drugs are good. Drugs are very, very good. For those of you who worry that I would get behind the wheel and drive myself to the doctor, don't worry; I was driven to the appointment by Ben Blake. I would never drive under the influence.

The walk from the parking garage to the doctor's office was something else. It felt like the death march on Bataan. With each step I repeated the same words, "And that bitch wanted me to go to Cedars to get blood drawn." I literally crawled up those stairs and down those halls with my Foley in a J. Crew bag. I was disguising it—or so I thought.

Then a man in his forties came up to me and said, "I'm getting that done next week."

"Congratulations." I said as sarcastically as I could.

He laughed, "Is it bad?"

"Ohhhhh noooo. Just slam your hand in a car door and you'll see what it's like."

Thank God he had a good sense of humor. He laughed. I told him it wasn't that bad and just to be prepared to not feel like himself. He had a thousand questions for me. I could see that he wanted some kind of insight into what he was about to experience. I wanted the same thing before my surgery and so I understood. I wanted someone to say, "Hey, it's nothing. You'll be up and about in twelve hours." That's what I wanted, but it's not what I got. I wanted to make sure this man had something to hang his hat on in terms of expectations. I told him that he will be exhausted, that he will be in some pain but the pain can be managed with pills and that he must have loving people around him to help him through the tough times. He thanked me and shook my hand. It was like we were in some kind of brotherhood, some fraternity of men who had no prostate or were about to have no prostate. This was a club of which I never wanted to be a member. We chatted a few more minutes then I wished him well and continued to crawl up the rest of the hall on my hands and knees screaming to the gods to make the pain stop (Interesting side note #212: I can get a little dramatic at times).

I finally make it up to the doctor's office where I am rushed into a private room. I guess they don't want potential patients seeing you ashen, gaunt, and unable to stand while carrying a J. Crew bag. It's probably bad for business. "He's not in to have his prostate removed is he?" and then the waiting room clears out in a stampede of screaming men with their wives. I get into the room as I wait for the big moment when I will be detached from my J. Crew bag. The nurse comes in to take my vitals. I recognize her voice as the person who had said, "No. We don't do that." To educate her and perhaps help the next patient I said, "In case it comes up again, Medicare will provide a home health nurse for blood draws and things like that. They come to the house and they are wonderful."

"Oh really." She said with a flippant I-don't-really-care tone in her voice and walked out of the room without a smile or concern that I could possibly fall over dead in the office.

My blood began to boil. I was having the worst week of my life and there is a nurse who could care less about me or the pain I'm going through. The good news is she was the only person at Cedars with that attitude. Everyone else, to a person, was incredibly compassionate and caring. When you go into a field like medicine it's because you care about others; but every so often someone goes in because they couldn't get into cosmetology school. I guess there has to be a bad apple in every bunch.

I reminded myself that I wasn't there to educate this woman, I was there to get the Foley taken out—so I focused on that. I dreaded the moment. In one of my plays, there's a line where a character is waiting for his judgmental mother to arrive; he's anxious and full of self doubt and says in reference to having to wait for his mother to arrive, "Now I know how Anne Frank felt." There was a tense knot in my stomach as I sat there with my eyes fixed on the doorknob, waiting for it to turn and for the doctor to enter. It seemed like he never was going to come.

It must have been four minutes before the doctor arrived; to me it was an eternity. I was really glad to see him. He is a wonderful doctor and very nice man. He asked me how I was doing. I told him I was fantastic and I was running a 10K tomorrow. Nothing. Didn't get the joke. He then went about looking at the incision and poking me here and there. Then suddenly the Foley was out. Huh? What just happened? I have to tell you, my doctor was a genius at removing Dr. Foley's little bit of magic tubing. My doctor had a little trick. He was talking to me and gesturing with his right hand. He had my full attention looking at his right hand, and while I was looking over here, he yanked the Foley out over there. He was like a magician using distraction to make his magic work. It was painless. Of course, the pain pills I had taken may have dulled the pain, but I wanted to think I had the best doctor in Los Angeles. Dr. Magic fingers, The Houdini of Foley removal. I wanted to be able to tell everyone, "I didn't feel a thing," but being a comedian I couldn't help myself. Right after her pulled the Foley out I said to him, "Did you ever do that and have a lawn mower start?"

He looked at me like I was insane. "Why would a lawn mower start from removing a Foley catheter?"

I began to explain it to him, stopped, and put my pants back on. Doctors. They have absolutely no sense of humor. I guess that's a good thing. You don't want them in the operating room cracking jokes, "How many surgeons does it take to remove a prostate?" You want him focused on what he's doing; but I'm a comedian—I am always looking for the laugh. I should have learned from the, "Bad dog. Bad dog!" joke I did a couple of weeks prior. However, I did manage to get a laugh out of him finally. In passing a friend mentioned to me that when he had the Foley taken out the doctor forgot to deflate the balloon and it was very painful. I said to the doctor, "I was told to remind you to deflate the balloon," and he laughed like it was a comedy club and I had just closed the show. For the life of me, I will never figure out what it takes to make this man laugh—and this is what I do for a living.

Anyway, the catheter is out. Then I learned from the doctor that I have a testicular infection. It's sort of a gift with purchase; remove one prostate, get one infection. Normal, I'm told. Maybe it's normal for *you*—not so normal for me. I'm put on a regimen of antibiotics. I add those pills to my daily regimen of painkillers, stool softeners, and laxatives. In the sixties I took drugs. Good drugs—drugs that had you laughing for hours. At my age, I've come to the full circle of drug use: stool softeners and laxatives. At least I'm here to complain about it; many of my friends are not. There was one thing about those antibiotics that I must tell you—they were the same size as the pills they gave to Secretariat. I had to break them in half to get them down and they still got stuck in my throat. I never have trouble taking pills, but these pills were impossible to get down. I want to sit in a room with the pharmaceutical manufacturer and say, "Go ahead, take one. I dare you," and laugh with glee as he chokes to death. I'm not being too dramatic, am I?

Now let me reflect on the good drugs I got in the hospital that first week. I was given Oxycodone every four hours. There were junkies in coffee shops in Amsterdam who were not taking their pills as regularly as I was taking mine. Along with the Oxy came the rest of the cocktail—stool softeners. I've heard about opioid constipation. Unless you've experienced the joy of opioid constipation, you don't know what fun is. Think about trying to shove a block of concrete through the eye of a needle. You know there is something there but it's at a standstill—lodged like the 405 Freeway at rush hour. You push (my hat is off to any woman who ever heard that word in a delivery room). You push, but your hernia doctor has told you to never push too hard because you could break the mesh from your hernia operation six months prior. That's another story for another day, another book (Interesting side note #569: You should see my stomach. It looks like the switching yard for the Union Pacific Railroad). I know why people are dying of opioid addiction—their intestines exploded. That's why I was determined to eat roughage. I was grazing roughage like Elsie the Borden's cow, but none of my efforts proved helpful. For five days there was nothing. Then, rumblings. I run to the bathroom and sit there like I'm waiting for the E Train in Manhattan going downtown. Twenty minutes later, I produce two raisinettes and something that looked like Streisand's profile. I didn't care. To me that was best movement I ever had. I was not adding constipation to my current list of ailments, which was already long and colorful. At the next office visit when the doctor asks if I am regular, I will say, "Yes, like clockwork." Screw 'em. I've got this totally under control. More flax seed?

After the Foley removal I leave the doctor's office like a bird who has flown the nest for the first time since emerging from the egg. I am free. I am no longer holding my J. Crew bag full of urine, and believe me J. Crew is happy about that. It can't be good for their business.

"What did you get at J. Crew?"

"A Foley Bag and some urine."

"Was that from their spring collection?"

"Oh yes, everyone will be wearing this next year."

The car is two stories down, then a fifty-yard walk to the parking garage, then up a slight inclined ramp to where it is parked. I make it two-thirds of the way to the car when suddenly, without warning, I just go completely limp. My legs give out from under me and I'm shuffling backwards like a tap dancer auditioning for *A Chorus Line* trying to regain my footing, but to no avail. I'm wobbling like the scarecrow in *The Wizard of Oz*. I could not grab hold of anything because there was nothing to grab hold of. I was in the middle of the parking ramp. I couldn't find the strength in my legs to stop the downward spiral and so I continued to shuffle backwards. Then, suddenly, I slam into a wall. It stops my inevitable drop to the floor and I'm able to push myself up to a semi-upright position. I grab on to the wall for dear life and just stand there for a moment. Cars are passing me by as they continue on their search for an open parking spot. No one is helping me because no one has seen my tumble and no one knows I'm in distress. I don't like that I'm in distress. I'm not a distress kind of person. I'm always in control. Today, as I lean against the wall in the parking garage, I feel like a hooker waiting for a John. Finally, out of nowhere, a hand reaches out to me. I looked at that hand with a great deal of gratitude because there was no way in hell I was going to be able to bring myself to an upright position. The stranger pulls me forward and into a standing position. He had witnessed my spiral down and had come over to lend a hand. He stands there for a second, "Are you ok?"

I nod. I thanked him and he went on his way. Every so often he would turn and watch me to make sure I wasn't going to fall again as I made my march to the car. The friend who had driven me to the appointment had walked ahead of me and was on a different level of the parking garage when I began to fall. He was going to get the car to bring it to me, so he didn't see my demise. In the past I would have been very angry that he abandoned me, but today I had no resentment for him leaving me. It's not his job to be my bodyguard. He was nice enough to drive me today. I said nothing as I got into the car. It was then I realized the surgery had changed me. It had truly changed me. I am grateful now for the little things like a stranger's helping hand, like a friend driving me to an appointment, like having the Foley out and knowing that I was one step closer to a recovery. I can no longer be upset by the little mishaps in life. My perspective is different now. Cancer has given me a whole new outlook on my life. I got into the car, smiled, and we headed home. I open the window so the breeze could keep me alert and so I don't pass out on Santa Monica Blvd—that's how exhausted I was. Yet despite the trauma, I am happy that I am alive and feeling better.

Feeling better—are there no nicer words? In that second week you think you are feeling better. You see, that's where they get you,

you *think* you're feeling better but you actually are not. You're able to get out of bed and walk to the kitchen with out much difficulty, but by the time you get there you need a wheelchair to get you back into bed. At this point I can't say I was in pain, I just wasn't feeling like my old self. I was just feeling old. I had stopped taking the painkillers in an attempt to have a bowel movement sometime prior to my death. No, pain was not the word I would use to describe what I was experiencing in that second week. What I was experiencing was complete and continuing exhaustion. It's the kind of exhaustion that makes your bones ache; the kind of exhaustion that makes you so tired you can't find a comfortable place for your head on the pillow. Your entire body pulses with a kind ache that you have never experienced before and hope you will never experience again. You want to just get into bed and relax, but you are just so uncomfortable it's not an option. The second week was not fun and anyone who tells you, "Hey, it's not so bad," can kiss my ass in Macy's window, as the expression goes.

There was one thing and one thing only that got me through that second week, and that was the love and support of my friends. Not my family, because those people ignored my surgery like it was an imposition on their time. I did not hear from one of them. That hurt so much because as a child, I was told, "The family will always be there." Now, that may have been a distortion of the reality, but it's what I believed all my life. Here I was, in need of them the most, and the silence was deafening. I did get a couple of emails from them— one that read, "Sorry you're going through this," and another that read, "This is what happens when you get to our age." The warmth of those emails couldn't fill a flea's navel, to borrow an expression said about William Morris agents. There were two bright spots: one, a cousin—the wife of a blood cousin—who did write and wrote with sincerity and with love and it was greatly appreciated because she was just what I needed when I needed it the most. The second, the daughter of a cousin who sent me one of those things that look like flowers but are actually cantaloupe. The rest of the family only proved what I had felt for decades: a cut off and self-involved group of people with which I had the unfortunate fate of sharing DNA.

It was my friends—my loving, generous, giving friends—that proved to me family doesn't have to be about blood, it can be about love. At one point I stopped and I looked around my room. It was filled with flowers and cards. There were balloons drifting about my head, and I had an epiphany. It was something that numerous shrinks had been trying to make me see for decades, I simply had not been able to see it. Cancer and prostate surgery opened my eyes; I finally got it. I finally got that people truly cared about me even if my family couldn't. I finally got that I was worthy. I finally got that what had been told to me all my life, that I was a selfish, ungrateful pig, was wrong. I am not a selfish, ungrateful pig. The realization overcame me in a quiet moment in my bedroom on that second week, and I broke down and cried. I was helped to that realization by looking at those flowers and get-well cards. It came from seeing enough food delivered to my house to feed Oprah's gratitude class. It came in the form of cakes and cookie baskets, muffin baskets, deli platters, and gallons of chicken soup—which was the only thing I could get down that second week. It was an outpouring of love that touched me to my very core. It helped me through the roughest week of my life and it changed my life.

While I held a resentment for family that didn't call, there were friends who were closer than family that also did not call. I had no ill feeling towards them. There was one person in particular, we are closer than family and they didn't come to visit or send a card or call in that first two weeks. I finally got an email saying, "I'm going to try to get up there." I know this person and I know how hard they work. Their life is consumed with work and helping others. When they are not rescuing animals they are rescuing people, and it's all they do. They have a heart of gold and I know it would be difficult to pull themselves away from their work to spend time with me. I gave them the best gift I could give. I said, "Look, I don't need you in the room to let me know you love me. I know you love me. So take 'visiting Steve' off your to-do list because you, above everyone else, don't have to show me you love me. I know you love me." We never spoke of it again. It made me feel so good to be able to do that for them. It made me realize once again that I was changing. I wasn't so needy. I was able to give back. It was a great feeling because it felt like growth, and growth is what you want when you reach my age. Actually, when you reach my age, being able to remember where you left your cell phone is a gift. I pride myself in continuously working on myself. When they finally lower me into the ground they will probably hear from inside the casket, "I get it. I finally get it."

When you're lying in bed and you have lots of time to think, you think. I tried to understand why I was able to give the gift of unconditional love to my friend who was so busy with her own life. The answer came back time and time again: I was able to give because the pain of my childhood was finally out of my life. I was able to forgive those that tortured me, that belittled me, that negated me, that neglected me, and I was able to move on. No longer did I have the empty feeling of there being someone out there who was supposed to love me unconditionally but wasn't able to. Once that burden was lifted from my shoulders, I was able to get out of myself and give to others. If those two weeks of pain and discomfort taught me anything, they taught me that. It's almost worth having prostate cancer... but the verdict is still out on that one. It's only the second week.

You see, I have always been someone who could never feel the love of others. I used to say the love stopped about a foot from my heart, but it never went inside to my soul. After the prostate surgery I could no longer say that. In the first two weeks, after I got home from the hospital, over twenty people came to visit me in my house. Twenty people left the routine of their daily lives to came to my house and sit on my bed to make me laugh or just tell me they loved me. By the third week that number had climbed to thirty-one people. This universal effort forced me to stop and look at who I was as a person and what impact I had on the people around me. I could no longer say I didn't matter to anyone. The outpouring of love that was given to me, was *that* overwhelming. I could no longer believe the inaccurate view my parents had of me. My parents saw me through the distorted glasses of their own troubled upbringing, of their own failures. They were unable to nurture, and it led me to believe that no one could ever care about me. I thought if my own parents were unable to give me what I needed, then who could? I mean, if your own parents can't care, there must be something really wrong with you. Through this ordeal I learned that this was my parent's problem, not mine. They were dealing with their own problems. The sad part of this scenario, none of this would have happened if my parents had not passed away—my dad first many years ago, and my mom just a few years ago. They would never have been able to see my reality as I am seeing it now. They just were never given the tools to see past their own problems, and because of it they were deep in denial. Sadly, their deaths freed me. It's a horrible thing to say, but it's the truth. Seeing me as I am today would have meant they were wrong, and they could never admit that. It just wasn't in their makeup. They had to die and free me so I could live.

The fact that I was loved by so many was made even more obvious by the actions of my college roommate from Emerson College, Bob Fisher. Bob lives on the east coast, so we really haven't spent any time together since college. First he moved to the Caribbean, then to New York City while I was on the west coast. Our lives took separate paths, but the emotional bond we had developed in college remained. We didn't need to be together to *be* together. That one year Bob and I spent together with our other roommate, Jon Stierwalt, in that tiny little college apartment on Warrington Street on a back street in Boston bonded us for life. A true brotherhood developed, and Bob Fisher showed that bond by calling me every day from the day I left the hospital till the day I said to him, "Bob, you are off support duty. I get it. You love me. And I love you. You no longer need to call me. I'm okay." I needed him to know I was on the mend and he could go on with his life with his wife. When you have a bond like that with someone, when they understand you like Bob understood me, it's better than if you were handed bricks of gold. Bob stopped the calls, but we don't need calls to love each other. That will always be there. It felt good that I could free Bob of his responsibility of calling me every day. It felt good that I could let him know that I felt his love and that it was mutual. That's what brothers do.

Jon Stierwalt was my other roommate when I lived with Bob Fisher. As close as Bob and I are, Jon and I had an even closer relationship. Jon was raised by a single mother. I was raised by a single mother. He never got laid in college. I never got laid in college. He had a wild sense of humor. I had a wild sense of humor. I loved Jon in a way that was different from Bob. Jon was Svengali—he could talk anyone into anything. It endeared him to me because back then, I was so shy. Jon made me laugh like no one could. Jon and I had stayed in touch more than Bob and I, if you think finally calling each other after twenty-five years is keeping in touch. When we did finally get in touch, it was like no time had passed. We simply picked up like we had just left our apartment on that back street, behind the Shubert Theater in a seedy part of Boston.

Jon had told me he was going to be out of the country in Colombia with his wife when I was having surgery, but he would call me the moment he got back. The day he landed in Miami he called to check up on me. He said, "I just needed to hear your voice. I just needed to know you were okay." It was the special bond that we share. I was an only child, but I have two brothers that are closer to me than blood brothers. It's a blessing I will always be grateful for.

Jon and I love to make each other laugh. I think he was the first to understand I had a natural ability for comedy, but on this phone call two weeks after prostate surgery, all I could do was cry with him. These were tears of joy. Tears because I finally could feel how Jon felt about me. How could I not have seen it? How could I have believed my parents' sick, demented view of me? Strangely enough, it took prostate cancer to make me understand it all. How could I not accept and feel the love that was being sent my way? The answer was, I couldn't, so the surgery has become a life-changing experience for me. It taught me that I could never again say, "I don't matter." I learned that I do matter.

That was Bob and Jon, my two brothers, fifty years later, and still checking up on me. How do you repay someone for that kind of devotion? You can't. You just accept it and make the devotion reciprocal. Bob and Jon—my brothers from other mothers—they were there during my transition from living at home to being on my own, they shared my life with me and continue to share it to this day. I am a very lucky man. There were many other special people.

Susan Salter Roderick and I grew up together in Boston. As luck would have it, we went to college together as well. It's amazing the kind of bond that is created at Emerson. It's like a mafia you can't get out of but actually want to stay in. Susan called a couple of times to check in on me and to tell me she loved me. It wasn't just that she called to tell me she loved me, it was the sincerity in her voice that made me understand. She truly cared and she told me how important I had been in her life. It was so strange to hear that since I never felt enough to be in anyone's life. Mom had done a hell of a job on my self worth. I learned that I have devoted friends because *I* am a devoted friend. It's nice. It's good. It's the way it should be—and if cancer had to teach me anything, it's taught me that.

That was the good stuff I remembered from the first two weeks after surgery, but let me tell you, it's not all a basket of roses and lollipops. There are a couple of thorns in there as well. I call them my friends that are not on my shit list, but who I'm putting on the "shit-list-adjacent" list. You see, I'm not angry enough at them for them to be on the shit list so it's to the "shit-list-adjacent" list they go. I will never abandon them no matter how crappy a friend they turned out to be—two wrongs don't make a right. As I write this, you will be happy to know that long after the two-week period, I have destroyed the shit-list-adjacent list and just accepted everyone for what they are able do or what they are not able to do. With some people you just can't ask them to give or understand or be empathetic, it's just not who they are. You know the animal and you put them in a place where their actions don't hurt you. Talk about growth!

There is one other group of people who will forever have a special place in my heart. These are people who came to the hospital to visit me the few days I was there. Parking at Cedars costs about as much as a two bedroom duplex in Manhattan (are you getting the point about me and paying for parking? The hospital is charging me $90 for a :d blanket, would it kill them to make parking reasonable?), but there were people who weren't concerned about the price of parking and showed up in my hospital room, like Randy Kirby, the funniest man in Los Angeles. Randy has been a friend for over forty years, like a brother. He came and spent only five minutes with me because I was just too exhausted to be a host. I felt horrible that I couldn't be more receptive to his visit, but the Oxy had just kicked in. His monumental effort to come see me where the parking office has an escrow department, earned him a special place in my heart for eternity. Then there's Paul Sanderson. Paul was a writing partner about forty years ago and showed up on the second day I was in the hospital. There I was lying in my hospital bed, bored, scared, tired, and suddenly the door opens and Paul walks in. My heart soared. I cannot tell you what Paul's visit meant to me in that moment. It was an act of love that only true friends share. Julie and Sam Bobrick came. I love them because no matter what the situation, Sam and Julie can find the funny in it, and we always end up laughing, which is what happened the day they showed up. Sandra J. Mendelsohn Brown, a Facebook friend, said she was coming up to the hospital, and she did. We really didn't know each other, but she made the effort to come see me, and now I will walk through fire for her. These are angels on earth whose capacity to love goes far beyond those of others and certainly make up for the shit-list-adjacent people in my life. Then there was Lynne Kuykendall; she was a complete stranger. I had never met her. I didn't know her. She didn't know me, but my friend of forty years, Sheila Washington, who lives in New York City, called her friend Lynne in Los Angeles and told her to go visit Steve in the hospital. And Lynne did. This charming, lovely, beautiful woman sat in my room and we talked like we had known each other for our entire lives. It was one of the most heart-warming experiences I had in the hospital. I was on my adventure into surgery and she came to help me through it.

I will carry with me forever the warmth of that visit. I think of all the visitors, I loved Lynne the most. This is someone who truly gives from the heart and gives to a stranger. We are strangers no more; we are now bonded in friendship though her act of kindness.

If we could only spread around a little of what was given to me. If the racists could only learn to accept, if the anti-Semite could see we are all the same, if people would just learn to love instead of hate—oh, who am I trying to fool? The world is a cesspool and we have to learn how to swim in it. But if just for a brief moment you are reminded of how good the world could be, well then maybe having your prostate ripped out of your body right in the middle of the holiday season could be worth it.

Week Three. Come On Let's Get Out of This Bed

This is the strangest week of all. Why? At this point you're not sick enough to stay in bed and yet not well enough to go out into the world. You're in the purgatory of recovery. You want to go out and boogie, but if you do you'll be back on the eighth floor at Cedars eating things that look like chicken but taste like inflatable tires. You try to do something productive with your time but as soon as you get started you're so tired your legs ache. When I say your legs ache, I mean they ache in a way you have never felt aching before. It's like they are on fire from the inside out. Nothing you do eases the ache. So, you crawl back into bed where you stay until you've had a three-hour nap. Before this surgery, I never napped. I was always too anxiety-driven to just sit and do nothing. I had to be doing something at all times to keep my mind occupied and off my feelings of failure. In week three, however, getting up to go to the bathroom had me napping for two hours. Going to the kitchen, one hour. I was thinking of putting a mobile over my bed like they do with infants.

I did try to do little things, things that wouldn't tire me out—like balancing my checkbook. The damn thing was $600 off. The bank said I had $600 less than I said I had in my account. In the past I would have gone through that statement with a fine tooth comb searching for that lost $600, trying to figure out how the bank had managed to steal that much money from my account without me noticing. I just know that the bank is out to screw me for my $600. They need my money, how else can they build those buildings on Wilshire? How else can they build those buildings in downtown Manhattan? The skyline of hundreds of cities is dependent on the money they steal out of my checking account. Usually I would have called and screamed until they gave me the $600 just to shut me up, but this time I just said, "Fuck it," and adjusted my checkbook down $600. It is what they call in AA a "surrender." I just didn't have the fight left in me to go to the mat for the money. Is my health worth $600? The answer was yes, so I surrendered and reduced my checking account balance $600 and then took a nap. The prostate won. I don't know if it was the anesthesia, the surgery itself, or that fact that every extra ounce of strength had been sucked out of me. I just didn't care. Let them keep my money. They must need it more than I do. Although that was before I saw the price of Depends. Why are adult diapers so expensive? Is Queen Elizabeth hand-knitting them?

The point I'm making is, see what the surgery has done for me? It's made me see life in a different light. Life is too short to let the little stuff bother you (see paragraph on the shit-list-adjacent people). You have to pick your battles. The bank is always right. In forty-five years of balancing my checkbook, not once have I caught the bank in a mistake. So relax, Steve, adjust your checkbook and live a few years longer. You probably forgot to enter a check for $600.00 anyway. You know you haven't been yourself lately. That's how I ended this little episode—not worrying about the $600. My close friends who are reading this just sat down and started to fan themselves (interesting side note #3358: two months after I deducted the $600 from my checking account, my checking account balance was over $600. You see, the Lord giveth and the Lord taketh away, and evidently so does Bank of America).

The wonderful thing about the third week is that the gifts of love still keep coming. One day the deli that's near my house wanted to know if I was going to be home. Yeah, like I could go out bloated the size of a Chris Christy doll, and with dripping diapers. Within the hour, two huge bags of food arrived at my house; Corned beef, Swiss cheese, rye bread, a gallon of chicken soup, a dozen black and white cookies. It wasn't a care package, it was a huge "I love you" wrapped in tin foil. You see, three friends I had made in New York City in the 1970s got together and sent me the gift of love. That's all I could call this wonderful surprise because that's what it felt like to me. We haven't lived close to each other for decades, yet the connection remains as close as it was when we all lived on East 58th street. I have to add, the gift of love came at exactly the right time. I had eaten almost everything that had been sent to me over those first three weeks. The gift of love replenished my supplies for another week, not only in the refrigerator, but also in my heart. Where do you find friends like this? I guess you find them in my life. Nice, isn't it?

The visits continued in the third week as well. The visits were more fun in the third week because I didn't keep falling asleep in front of the visitors. I was able to laugh with them and talk with them and tell stories and genuinely be a host. I loved it, and more importantly I loved that my friends took time out of their day to come to my home and show me they cared. I couldn't believe they actually cared about me, but they did. The surgery had become a massive learning lesson, and each day I was using that lesson to shake myself out of old habits learned. This lemonade from lemons thing became a mission. I could no longer deny my place in the world. My friends would not let me.

Oh but wait, there's more news. In week three I made my first venture out into the world. That's right, prostate boy was leaving the house. It was now November and Christmas was looming on the horizon. I needed cards. I needed wrapping paper. I needed to buy gifts, but how could I do all that in my present condition? I asked a friend to take me to the 99 Cent Store. Oh shut up, it was close to the house and I could be down another $600 in my checking account at any moment.

Going out into the world after you have had major surgery is truly a fascinating experience. No one knows you've just had surgery and they continue on their lives like normal. But you, you are moving like a snail on Medicaid and they don't know why you are protecting your groin with both hands. I'll tell you why. Every shopping basket that passes is a potential groin-piercing missile. Every child running across the room with flailing arms becomes a dagger soon to be inserted into your intestine. Every large dog that wants to shove his nose into your crotch becomes a pack of ravenous wolves looking for vulnerable prey. I have never been more fearful of my life than I was at the 99 Cent Store. Look, the 99 Cent Store is a freak show on a regular day, but add my present condition to it, and it becomes an episode of *American Horror Story*. I couldn't wait to get out of that snake pit. I got my wrapping paper and fled for my life (interesting side note #999: I love asides—it's so Shakespearian. When I started writing the Christmas cards that I bought at the 99 Cent Store I was able to see them in the right light for the first time. I was able to see that they were so old they were starting to yellow. Did I care? No. I have no prostate anymore. I sent the cards with my signature and a little note: "ONLY THE FINEST THE 99 CENT STORE CAN OFFER").

I had the cards and wrapping paper covered by the 99 Cent Store, but what about the gifts? I was perplexed as to how I was going to get to Macy's and fight the crowds with no prostate. Then, like some divine intervention from above, I heard this word ring in my ears— Amazon! At first I thought to myself, *I'm not going to Brazil to go Christmas shopping.* Then it hit me—Amazon.com—the world of shopping at your fingertips. There is a god! I crawled up to my office and sat myself down in front of my computer with my Christmas list and a wireless mouse. Within one hour I had purchased everything. Two days later it arrived at my front door. It's like the miracle at Lourdes. Ask and ye shall receive. Only in this case, it's click and they will deliver—as long as you have a working credit card. Another lesson learned; for every problem there is a solution.

Oh! I almost forgot, there was one more miracle. In the third week, I made the bed. Now, that's no big deal for a lot of you, but for me it was huge. For three weeks the bed has been left unmade with the comforter piled up in the corner of the room. It sort of looked like a high-end homeless person was living there. No big deal for most people, but for me it was a majorly big deal. I'm anal-retentive with OCD tendencies—everything must be in its place at all times. It comes from a childhood trauma of being left homeless with my mother after she divorced my father. Since the day we came home to learn my father had moved and given up our apartment, leaving my mother and I with no place to live, I always have to know where my possessions are at all times and they have to be in order and organized. That pile of bedding was driving me crazy, so three weeks into my prostate vacation I was strong enough to get out of that bed and make the bed the way it was supposed to be, God damn it!!! No longer would the comforter be piled up in the corner. It has found it's home on the bed looking like the front page of the Ballard Designs Catalogues.

I could no longer recuperate by lying around in the bed all day. It was official. I was on the mend, and making the bed was the first indication of that. It's these little milestones that bring such joy to a person when one is inching his was back to health free of prostate cancer. Free of prostate cancer, are those not the most wonderful words you have ever heard? I am free, wow! I am well aware that ten to thirty percent of men experiencing prostate cancer will have a reoccurrence. At this very moment, however, my doctor told me, "Steve, you are cancer free," and since I live in the moment, for today I am cancer free. And my bed is made. It's a double miracle. Thank you Jesus (or whoever you chose to thank).

Week Four. Look Out World Here I Come... Sort of

In the fourth week, things started to kick up a notch. I started to go out of the house. I went to Costco, and it almost killed me. Costco when you're feeling fit-as-a-fiddle is a nightmare with the crowds fighting for free samples and you trying to lift a fifty-pound bag of dog food, but four weeks after major surgery adds a whole new fear to the experience. I had to go, though, because there was no food in the house. It was either go to Costco or start eating small bits of the furniture. I wasn't looking forward to it. Every rushing person was a threat to my ability to stay upright. At one point I just had to pull myself out of the flow of traffic and grip on to a fifty-pound box of Depends. Depends, there you are, my new best friend! As if having prostate surgery is not bad enough, now you have to wear diapers out in public. My friend Carol says, "Don't say diapers. Say pull-ups." Yeah, cause there's such a big difference between diapers and pull-ups. What does it matter, I'm peeing in my pants in either case. Ugh! This after-affect of wearing pull-up diapers (Happy Carol?) is the added insult to injury. You are left incontinent—and when I say incontinent I don't mean I'm spending the summer in Europe. I mean your new best friend is a box of super-absorbent cotton humiliation pants, because when you stand, you pee. When you cough, you pee. When you pee, you pee. How could this happen to a nice kid like me? I had not planned for this in my retirement. I was going to wear Speedos to the beach. The only way I can wear a bathing suit to the beach now is if it has a skirt. Oh yeah, and you think a box of Depends is cheap? A box of Depends costs $43. $43 for paper underwear that makes it impossible to get into any of your pants because of the bulk they add to your butt. Wearing adult diapers—because that's what they are, I don't care what their marketing department or Carol calls them, they are diapers—is an experience I wish on no one. Having no control of your bladder is another new experience I don't wish on anyone. Wait. There is one comedian who I hate. Him, I wish them on. I was warned by several of my friends what to expect, but until you actually experience the sensation of peeing in your pants, there is no way to explain the joy of incontinence. Sounds like a new self-help book. The Joy of Incontinence: Get to know what wet is. Just know that if you are not peeing in your pants without any control, you're a winner (interesting side note #705: I got hand-me-down Depends. A friend's father had just passed away from Alzheimer's. I got his leftover Depends. Another friend who just had the same surgery came over with his leftover diapers. When I was a child I got my cousin's hand-me-down underwear. His name was Harvey but written in the underwear was the name Michael, so I was getting hand-me-downs that were hand-me-downs. I thought I would never have to live that experience again, but here I am as an old man getting hand me down Depends).

In week four, I was using five diapers a day. I couldn't just go out of the house, I had to have something to carry my supplies in. I started calling my briefcase "the diaper bag." I couldn't be out of the house for more than two hours, otherwise my diapers became so heavy I started to walk like a drunk toddler. By the way, I take my hat off to those little cockers. They are learning to walk and getting their balance while caring around three pounds of pee. Those children are miracles, because one pound of wet diaper and I'm a blabbering idiot. Those kids are managing what a grown adult can't do. I walk like I'm carrying around a beach ball between my legs. I am so slow octogenarians are yelling at me to get out of the way. My biggest obstacle was the constant fear that I may appear wet and that my diapers might leak through my pants. I was constantly touching my ass to test for dryness, which really went over well in line at any grocery store. "Hey, do that at home pervert," says the lady standing behind me in line.

Did you know there is a diaper etiquette? You just can't change your diaper when you're out and leave it in somebody's bathroom wastebasket. You have to bring supplies with you. This includes plastic bags, powder, and additional diapers. When Ringling Bros. went on the road, they didn't bring as much crap as I had to bring when I left the house. Have you ever seen a new mother with her diaper bag and all the accouterments that goes along with a newborn? That was me just leaving the house to meet someone for lunch. Every time I left the house Johnson and Johnson stock went up.

Here's a perfect example of what it was like in week four. It's Thanksgiving and I'm on my first official social outing after surgery. This is the first time I've been out in public with my diapers and diaper bag and walking like somebody's grandfather. Costco and the 99 Cent Store don't count—I didn't know those people. This was the first time out with friends and West Coast family, the good family. The hostess sits me next to the oldest man at the table who also has had prostate cancer, "So the two of you will have something to talk about over dinner." This will be an interesting conversation.

"So how's your erectile dysfunction?"

"Fine, how's yours. Can you pass the peas?"

"Oh, I've been passing the peas for weeks now," says I.

The dinner goes along nicely, I make it through to dessert and stay the appropriate time before I can flee for my life into dry clothing. I make a pitstop before I make the hour ride home. I dutifully put the old diaper in the plastic bag I've brought and stuff it in the diaper bag—I mean briefcase. As I'm saying my good byes and walking out the door, someone asks me to help them out to the car with their portion of their leftovers. Why do people come to dinner and take home leftovers? Do they want to continue eating in the car going home? Are they going to put them in their scrapbook? "Thanksgiving 2017. Giblets." I simply do not know why anyone takes food from a house where you have just eaten. Anyway, I help her into her car with her stuff, wave goodbye to the host and hostess, get in my car and head out for the one hour drive back home.

I'm home. I change my diapers and look for the powder, but it's not in the closet. Of course not, it's in my diaper bag, and my diaper bag *is in the bathroom of the house I just left.* Oh my god, there's a wet diaper in there! It's going to smell like the Gettysburg battlefield if that bag is not emptied. Now I have call and ask that question of the host, "So, did I leave my briefcase there? ...I did? ...Okay listen, it's too late to get it now...but... you're gonna have to open it and throw out the plastic bag that's inside. Either you do that or I'm gonna have to pay to have your bathroom repainted."

The host assures me it's no problem, but I know when he hung up the phone he turned to his wife and said, "That asshole left his dirty diapers here."

The next day I'm in my car making the two hour round trip to get my dirty laundry. I can't even begin to tell you what the feeling was walking into that house again. There I was, keeping up a brave face while dying of embarrassment on the inside. There are so many levels to the experience having prostate surgery. It's not just the surgery you have to deal with, it's the readjustment of learning how to live your new life. I'm doing my best at four weeks to make that adjustment, but it's no bed of roses, trust me.

Oh yes, did I forget to tell you I'm driving? The fear that had built up inside me of getting behind the wheel was overwhelming. I had not been in my car for five weeks. I was not as strong as I was. I was not as sharp as I was. I wasn't sure that when I got behind the wheel I'd be able to control the car, but I had to face my fears and drive. I backed that car out of the garage like it was loaded with nitroglycerin. I think it took me twenty minutes to get down the driveway, but I made it. I pulled out into traffic, and suddenly I had not been laid up in bed for four weeks. I was back behind the wheel without any fears at all. Strange how the mind works—until a car pops out from a driveway and I almost had a heart attack. Four weeks ago I would have rolled down my window and given him the finger. Today I am shaking like a leaf. The surgery has taken its toll, not only physically but emotionally. Like every other emotional battle I've had to fight in my life, I will get through this one with my own inner strength and the help of State Farm.

Weeks Five, Six, Seven and On to Infinity. It's the Neverending Story

At this point in recovery, you are on emotional hold. Things happen, but you are not aware they are changing for you. For instance, I ran up the stairs. That's right, I ran up the stairs. Didn't think about it. Didn't think that five weeks prior I had been so weak climbing those very same stairs that I had to have someone lend me support or else I'd have fallen backwards to a painful death (interesting side note #340: that would have so made me angry, to go through this surgery and die on the steps of my own home. What a waste of a perfectly good Foley Bag). Nope, I just bolted up the stairs, yet when I got to the top I did stop for a split second and relish in my miracle. That's what it's like in recovery, little miracles and little set backs. Here's some wisdom from the master of prostate surgery recovery: the body doesn't heal in a straight line. Your stomach will be flat as a board on Monday and you'll look pregnant on Wednesday. You'll be pain free on Tuesday and have pain on Thursday. You'll sleep like a baby on Saturday and be up all night on Sunday. It's a constant battle of up and down, forward and back, back and forward. You want there to be no backwards but there always will be. The thing to remember is it's always a slow progression forward in tiny increments. You may not feel it because it's a slow progression forward—a progression which will eventually bring you back to your old life. Remember this little bit of advice, because it will make you feel like there is some hope when you're sure there is none. You will be reminded that someday, someday in the near future, you will be able to be your old self again. There is always that moment of fear when you think that *this* may be your new self. That in five years you'll look back at this time period and say, "Remember when all I did was pee in my pants? I'm still doing that." You can't think like that, you have to take your recovery one day at a time and live for today. Today I am progressing nicely even if I don't see the progression. Now, if you'll excuse me, I'm going to change my diaper.

That's the worst adjustment, the incontinence. I am one of those immaculate anal-retentive people who must have everything in order, neat and clean at all times. The thought that I'm walking around in pee-soaked diapers has been the worst of the worst for me. I am always worried that I smell. I am constantly asking anyone around me, "Do I smell like a dog run?" I never do, but I am always afraid I do. It's one of the joys that came with this major surgery. When you're planning your surgery, you don't think about the period of recovery. You are consumed with the pre-operative stuff. The tests and the test results and making sure everything is in order before you go under the knife; but now all that stuff is behind you and you are forced to deal with the day-to-day of recovery and learning you are not the same person you were before you had prostate cancer. Things have changed in your life and you have to learn how to deal with them.

When I first decided to have this surgery, I truly didn't think of the consequences. My only thought was, *Get this cancer out of me as fast as you can*, and that's what they did. I am cancer free for now. I must say that time and time again to myself to keep reminding myself of the reality. I am cancer free for now. I don't have to worry that the pain in my back or the pain in my side is the cancer spreading. They got it all. There is a price to pay for that serenity: I'm walking around in pee-soaked diapers that limit my ability to be truly free. Some would say it's a small price to pay, but unless you've walked through the world fearing everyone is looking at you because your pants are wet, you don't know what hell is.

There are days when I just want to scream at the top of my lungs, "I'm so sick of this shit. When is it going to end??" Then I remind myself of what I have been through, take off the Depends, and put on a new pair of paper undies. Paper undies, it's a new fashion trend for the infirm. Maybe it'll catch on and all the kids will start wearing them to the beach—then I'll be hip again. That and many other things will never happen. I have to face it. It's a huge surrender on my part. A huge giving it up to a higher power that I know knows more than I do. I don't want you to think that I'm some kind of religious freak. I am not. I have been anti-religion since the age of eleven. However, I'm not anti-God. I'm anti-old men walking around in fancy clothes telling me they can talk to God for me, but that's a whole different book.

Now that I'm thinking of it, there is another side affect from the surgery that I have avoided speaking of like the plague. I don't want to think about it. I don't want to even pretend I'm thinking about it. It's the second whammy you get with the prostate surgery and it strikes at the heart of every man who has ever had this surgery. Impotence. I don't think there's a man alive who doesn't align his masculinity with the ability to have an erection. Well, that joy was taken away from me right after the surgery. On Monday you're a he-man. The day after surgery you're someone's great-grandfather who drools on himself. It's yet another gift-with-purchase that I didn't want.

When I first met with the doctor he explained to me that if the cancer had spread outside the prostate and into the area of the nerve bundle, he would have to cut the nerve and that would mean the end of erections for the rest of my life. Of course there were alternatives to solve that problem. There was the pump, however, I couldn't see myself blowing myself up every time I wanted to get intimate. I'd feel like some guy with a flat tire pulling into a gas station to get a little air from the air pump and we all know how well that worked out for me. Not well. There were alternative measures. For instance, I could inject myself with a needle in my private parts. When the words came out of the doctor's mouth my entire body went into organ rejection. A needle? There? Who thought of this, Mengele? No, that was not for me. I have to get a lollipop after my flu shot (Interesting side note #2014: my internist is also a pediatrician. When I do get a flu shot I actually *do* get a lollipop, but my favorite is the dinosaur Band-Aid. I just love that). There isn't a candy bar big enough to console me after injecting my manhood with a needle. Oh my God!!! Just writing those words, I want to crawl up into a ball and whimper like a puppy. There was one more alternative.

There were drugs that would help, the miracle drugs Viagra and Cialis. I wasn't opposed to that, after all, I had taken more drugs in the 1960s than Pfizer had produced in North America. I wasn't opposed to the idea of taking more drugs—until I called my insurance company. A three-month supply of either of these drugs was $6,800. In some countries that's a three-bedroom house. I don't care how much I wanted to feel masculine. I wasn't paying $6,800 every three months just to feel like Tarzan. I had to console myself that I just might have to live a life of solitude and limp celibacy. As one doctor put it, "At your age how many more erections do you think you're going to have?" That is the kind and sensitive doctor I did *not* let do the surgery.

There are alternatives to getting your drugs in the United States. When I was out and about having lab tests etc. and complaining about the costs of drugs in the United States, a lovely young lady sitting at a counter in one of the doctor's offices slid a piece of paper across the counter like we were having an affair and this was her phone number. I was half right—it was a phone number, but not for her. It was for a pharmacy in Canada. That explains why she handed that slip of paper to me like we were exchanging cash for a meth deal. You know, looking over your shoulder and sliding the paper across the counter like it was radioactive. I had never heard of such a thing, a pharmacy in Canada? I mean I know they had them, I just didn't know I could order from them. At the time, I did not know that it was frowned upon by the FDA and the drug industry in the United States. I just assumed that if a doctor's office slid me the piece of paper it must be okay. Stupid, uninformed me went for it hook, line, and sinker. I made the call. Yes, they had my drug. Yes, they could ship it to me. Yes, a three-month supply was $98. My first thought, *What's in it, Clorox and kitty litter?* I was assured that it was the same drug made under the same standards that any drug I could get in the States was made. That led me to my next questions: how fast can I get it, and why are drugs so expensive here in the United States? Why are people dying because they can't afford their meds and CEOs of drug companies are getting thirty million dollar bonuses? It angered me. I am a rebel. I rebel against injustice. I placed the order and gave the finger to the drug companies. I can see myself in jail.

"What are you in for?"

I bite on a toothpick hanging out of the side of my mouth and say, "Cialis."

I had to fax them the prescription and write them a check and fax the check and swear on a Bible that if I told anyone, they would come down to Los Angeles and repossess my erection. I agreed. The wheels were in motion for my illegal order. About four weeks later I got an email as they tracked my drugs.

"Your prescription is in Calcutta."

Then, "Your prescription was in Berlin."

"Your prescription is in Paris."

"Your prescription is in New York."

This shit traveled further than I did on the year I went to Europe after my college graduation (interesting side note # 12: I have not taken the medication. I couldn't get myself to take it. It was at this point that the doctor told me I wouldn't need it. The tumor had not grown outside the prostate and the nerve bundle was intact. Thanks. Great news, now that I'm a felon.)

Okay, so you have to know going into this whole surgery thing what the consequences might be. I knew what they were, but I still wasn't prepared to accept them, because those things just don't happen to me. As I waited for the lab results right after the surgery, my fears grew. When I got the call from my doctor, I almost burst into tears, "Steve, the lab results are back. The margins are clear. The lymph nodes are clear. The cancer was contained within the prostate. We got it all." He was kind and eloquent as he read the report to me. I could hear in his voice that he was happy for me. He told me that since the cancer had been contained within the prostate he didn't have to cut into the nerve bundle, but all I heard was, "You're going to have a hard-on again." My next internal question, *When?*

Despite the fact that everything points to me returning to normal within the year, the impatience is a motherfucker. There is always that voice in the back of your head that says, "What if he was wrong?" Those "what ifs" will kill you if you let them. You just have to let time take its course and let your body heal at its own pace. I'm doing that, but I'll be the first to tell you it's not easy. It's not easy to wonder what the rest of your life is going to be like. It's not easy to suddenly realize that despite the fact that you feel twenty-eight on the inside, you are seventy-one on the outside. It's not easy to see your friends die of one disease after another or have hip replacements or heart transplants or anything that comes with age. It's just not easy, and the reality that I'm facing is that I have aged and the best part of my life is behind me. It's not an easy pill to swallow, but at least it's a pill that's legal and I can get here in the United States.

You think having surgery like prostate surgery is a simple thing. You go into the hospital and they take it out. What you don't realize is how much this surgery effects your everyday life. It makes you stop and take an inventory of where you've been and what you've done. It also makes you think about your future and how you're going to use it. I've gotten a big fat dose of "Life is too short and it's time to live." When in the past, I may have said, "No, I'm going to wait until I'm older." Now I've realized, *I am older*. I've realized that if I don't start enjoying my life from this moment on, I'm going to end up one of those miserable old men yelling at the kids to get off his lawn. However, in my case it's miserable old man yelling at delivery trucks to get out of my driveway. We all dance to a different drummer. This is the time of your life when every minute counts and you have to take advantage of it. I am planning on doing that.

The Three-Month
Appointment Comes...Sort of

For three months I have been thinking of nothing else but my prostate and my recovery. The thoughts that go through my mind are endless. I am constantly questioning myself—is this normal, is that normal, am I healing at the proper rate of speed? Why does my pee smell like rotten eggs and sulfur? Did they take out my prostate and put in Satan? That can't be normal. You obsess and obsess and self diagnose but you're not a doctor and you don't know if you're on track or if you're the one who will be written up in *The New England Journal of Medicine*. You wait for the three-month appointment to find out how you're doing and it never comes. The days drag on like you're on death row. You try to find something to do; to pass the time you watch every movie you've ever wanted to see. You read. You reorganize your sock drawer. Twice. The three-month appointment never comes. Then, suddenly, you are about to go on that three-month visit to the doctor to see how *he* thinks you are doing. It's a scary yet happy appointment. I know I'm doing okay, but now I need him to tell me I'm doing okay. I never look forward to going to the doctors'—every time I go they find something new. It's part of the aging process. You go in for an earache he discovers your bowels are obstructed. How does that happen? It's like the car dealership that always finds something else wrong with your car. The radio doesn't work and they say you need a new transmission. This appointment has been three months in the making and I'm anxious to get it over with. I want to move on to the next stage of recovery. All I need is to hear from him is, "You're Fine."

I made my post-operative visit prior to surgery in October. I picked an easy date on the twenty-seventh. It was a Tuesday, a good day for me. I'm not a Monday person. I can't do anything on a Monday. Why? It comes from thirty-five years of being on the road and returning home on a Monday. Monday is the day I get to myself after traveling. It's my unwinding day, my stay home and pay the bills day and I never make plans on a Monday if I can help it. In any case, I have my Tuesday appointment and I'm ready to go.

Then that thing happens that always seems to happen to me happened. About two weeks after I made my office visit I get a call from the doctor's office.

"Mr. Bluestein, I'm sorry but the doctor isn't going to be here on the twenty-seventh."

"Ok, when does he want to see me?"

"How's the fourteenth?"

"Sounds good to me. It's an earlier date" (Valentine's Day). I'm good to go—again. The new visit is planned and without too much trouble or trauma. I'm a happy camper.

Like everything else in my life, nothing comes easy. That thing that always happens to me happened again. On about the seventh I get a phone call from the doctor's office.

"Mr. Bluestein. I'm sorry but I made a mistake. The doctor is not here on the fourteenth."

I think to myself, *Does he have a second job? Why is he never there? Maybe he's delivering pizzas for Pizza Hut. I mean, he has to practice medicine some time. Why can't I get one of those times? Why can't it be the fourteenth?* I quietly say to the young lady, "Ok, when can I see him?" When I say quietly, it was the kind of quiet that happens right before the volcano erupts or the tornado comes plowing through your barn.

"The sixteenth..." and I'm thinking that's not too bad. Only two days wait, "Of April" she says as sweetly as a judge sentencing a felon to death row. There is dead silence on my side of the phone.

Then, "Absolutely unacceptable! This is my three-month follow up visit after surgery. I had cancer. I am not coming in for an ingrown toenail treatment. I am not waiting until next April. That's two months away. Not waiting!!! Do you hear me?? Not. Waiting!" I scream.

"Well I'll let you talk to the office manager." she says as if she's talking to her mentally slow cousin.

This attitude angers me even more. She has made the mistake of twice scheduling an appointment when the doctor was not there and now expects me to put my anxiety on hold for two months while she does her nails or whatever the hell she does when she should be making office appointments for neurotic patients who have just had cancer surgery. "Right! Let me talk to the office manager!" I said sternly so she would know I was not happy. I was not getting off the phone until I had an earlier date for the next visit.

The office manager and I have a great rapport. Whenever she asked for something, like a blood test or an X-ray, I got on it as soon as possible. She answered every one of my neurotic emails. She listened to every insane question, "Will I be able to play the piano again?" She held my hand because this was a big step for me, and I needed to make sure that every "I" was dotted and every "T" crossed. She understood me and my anxiety, and she made the pre-surgery routine happen for me without a hitch. I made sure I sent her a Christmas gift just to make sure she knew how grateful I was for her kindness. Some people would say, "She was only doing her job," and that may be true but she did her job with grace and kindness. It's people like that you have to honor so they know they are appreciated. You see, her help made my journey possible. More importantly, this woman gets me and my anxiety, so I love her. Needless to say, after talking with her I'll be seeing the doctor on the fourteenth. The girl that had called me was mistaken… he *will* be in the office that day (I guess Pizza Hut is closed on the fourteenth). Oh! Don't you worry, I've already bought the candy for the office manager. She has saved my life once again. Good deeds must be rewarded. I am happy to reward them.

I wondered if it was only me that had problems with office staff like I was having, so I started asking around. As luck would have it, I have two friends going through the same prostate surgery. What do you mean, as luck would have it? Some luck. "Hey, you've got prostate cancer and you can take two friends along with you. And the winners are…"

I called the first guy. Nope, all his appointments were set and he's seeing the doctor on the appointed time. In all truthfulness, though, this is the same guy who had the surgery before me and said, "You'll be achy for a couple of days and you'll take pain pills. Then you'll switch to Tylenol and you'll be fine." I don't know what surgery he had, but the one I had kept me flat on my back for four weeks. He was right about the pain pills though. After the third day there was no need to take them. I was too constipated to worry about surgical pain and too tired to lift a glass of water to my lips to wash them down. That's the first of many lessons I learned from this dear friend, who is like a brother. Every person experiences prostate surgery differently. He had his experience. I was having mine. It wasn't fair to ask him how I was going to weather the surgery. Everyone's body is different. I'm an idiot for expecting our journey to be the same. Lesson one: everyone experiences the surgery differently.

I called the other friend and he said, "My doctor is a pig. His office looks like the food fight scene in Animal House. There are files stacked up on the floor and the office hasn't been cleaned since Roosevelt was in office. Teddy Roosevelt."

Okay, now we're getting somewhere. "Does he keep his appointments?" I ask with glee.

"Oh yes, and he's always on time."

Like I said, everyone has his own experience going through this. By the way, that friend switched doctors and is much happier with his new surgeon because his office was immaculate. This cancer thing is a nightmare to go through, but at least if you have friends to go through it with you to make you feel better (or worse) about your experience, you won't feel so alone. I suggest you start hanging out with smokers!

Then that thing that happens to me happened again. It's six days before my appointment on the fourteenth. At 4 p.m. I get a call. I see the caller I.D. it's my doctor's office and I answer the phone expecting the worst, "You're not going to change my appointment again, are you?"

"Oh no, Mr. Bluestein, I was just wondering if you had the PSA test?"

"What PSA test?"

"Oh the doctor needs you to have a PSA test before he sees you and it takes seven days to get the results."

"It's six days to my appointment! When were you going to tell me this? When I'm sitting in the waiting room??"

Silence.

I get the name of a lab and get up at 8 a.m. on a Saturday. Actually, I got up at 4 a.m. because I was so anxious about missing the blood draw appointment. I get to the blood draw appointment and then I learn that the orders for this blood work had been placed *last November.* They had two months to call and tell me I needed this test but waited till 4 p.m. on a day that was less than seven days before my appointment. I was livid on the inside but charming on the outside. The office worker at the lab asks, "This order was placed in November, why are you having it done so late?"

I answered with a smile on my face, "They just told me I needed this test last night. If they had trained apes in that office it would be more efficient." It's 9 a.m. and I got my first laugh of the day.

Then that thing happens that always seems to happen to me. I am told "Insurance will not cover this."

"Why?" I say through my gritted teeth.

"They used the wrong code for insurance and Medicare has rejected it."

At this point I realize that I am lucky to still be alive. The doctor is magnificent; his office staff came to this country on the Ship of Fools. I know what I have to do. I have to talk to the office manager, who I learn is out of the office for the next three hours. This is my major, big time, surrender for that day. I give the blood. I get back to my car and go home to watch MSNBC so I can vent my anger on Trump.

Three hours pass and I call the office. The office manager picks up the phone. I tell her today's dilemma and she says, "I know just what to do. I'll correct the code and you should be good to go." She is the only person in that front office who can hold an intelligent conversation, who is efficient, and who can solve my problems. If those other people only knew how their actions effected a patient they would.... Nah, nothing would change. They don't care. They're only there for the paycheck. It's the people like the office manager who do care that are the saving grace in a situation like this.

And so, as the sun sets in the west, we wait for next Wednesday and my visit with the doctor. My journey is almost over.

Oh really? The journey is almost over, huh? Honey, it's just begun. That thing that always happens to me happened again. I came down with the flu three days before the appointment. Let me repeat that. I came down with the flu three days before the appointment! Sore throat, body aches, headaches, coughing, spitting up things that looked like art installations; but all through it I kept saying, "I can still make the appointment." We can add dementia to that list of ailments I am left with. Finally I gave in, called the office and tell them I am too sick to see the doctor. I think that's an oxymoron—how can you be too sick to see a doctor? In this case, it was a reality. I was literally too sick to get out of bed to see him. They made me a new appointment. Sit down. Are you ready? May 9th. Ha!April doesn't seem too bad now does it, White Boy?

On the positive side, the blood test came back and my PSA was undetectable. This is exactly the result you want after you have prostate surgery. As of today, I am coughing my lungs out and being grateful that my blood test was perfect. Having prostate surgery was only the first step in a many-level process to complete recovery. The road is always filled with bumps and turns. You have to be able to roll with the punches, because the punches are many and they hurt. Take the small miracles when they come. Here's one. I am down to one diaper a day. Yippee! Whoever thought that would be a miracle? Dear Diary, I'm down to one diaper a day; let's go out and celebrate. I would, but I'm out of diapers.

I have mentioned the diapers several times because I detest them. We've discussed that they are a constant reminder that I am not well. They tie me down to the house because I'm afraid to go out in public with leaking pants and smelling like a homeless person. I'm always afraid I smell. I carry Febreze with me in the travel size, "For that personal odor problem." It's a horrible way to live. I am always afraid someone is talking about me behind my back. "Did you see the guy with the wet stain?" It's all in my mind because they don't leak. I have discussed all of this before, but it's really an issue with me. The diapers are also bulky and as ugly as a gorilla in a wedding dress. Another added attraction: they're impossible to get into because they collapse onto themselves as you put your foot into them. It's like they are fighting you and reminding you, if you were well, this wouldn't be a problem. The only good thing about them is that they are basically undetectable to the outside world.

The burning question that lives inside me, to the maker of Depends, is about the color. Grey? That's the color you came up with, industrial grey? What, did they have a sale on the paint lot? You had the entire color spectrum to pick from, and grey is what you decided everyone wanted. It's not reassuring. It makes you feel like you're a battleship in the Navy and getting ready for war. All it needs is "U.S.S. SARATOGA" on the side to make it "that perfect ensemble for any fall function." Oh yes, and they are expensive. Even at Costco. Then again, *everything* is expensive at Costco. I've saved so much money there now that I can't pay my mortgage, but these Depends are a whole new kind of expensive. There's sixteen cents of absorbent material, six cents worth of fabric-ish material to keep it all together, and some plastic cover that makes your butt sweat like you're running the Boston Marathon. Total output of these materials, twenty-two cents, which they are selling for about $2 each and insurance doesn't cover them. Which brings me to another story you won't believe.

I get in the mail an advertisement, "No more paying for diapers. Medicare will cover the costs. Just call us." I call them and I am told, "You never have to use diapers again. We have a new procedure and it's covered by insurance. What we do is glue the tip of your penis closed."

Hold it, "You glue the tip of my penis closed?"

"Right"

"Where does the urine go?"

"Out the side"

"Out the side of *what?*"

Long silence.

"I'm not interested." I hang up. I then wonder how many guys actually fell for this and got their penises glued shut. Barnum was right, there is a sucker born every minute. I want to state equivocally right here and now—no one is gluing the tip of my penis shut. Thank you!

The Setback Comes and It's a Big One

Everything had been going so well. I was down to one diaper a day. There it is again, me mentioning the diapers. Ugh. I was doing my Kegel exercises every day, four or five times a day. I did them in the car, I did them on the sofa, I did them with green eggs and ham. It was Kegel-mania over here at my house. For those of you who don't know this, there are Kegel exercises for men. The same exercises women use to strengthen the muscles that control the flow of urine are used for men. Women know what I'm talking about, but the first time it was mentioned to me I had no idea what a Kegel was. I thought it was one of those Russian pastries I grew up eating as a snack, "Come, Stevie, you'll have a Kegel and a glass tea."

It was all going great. Then I got the flu. I was flat on my back and sick as a dog. The last thing on my mind was my Kegel exercises. I was just trying to get air in and out of my lungs. The flu left me with bronchitis. The bronchitis left me coughing and choking at all hours of the day and night. It was an effort just to breathe and little by little the Kegel exercises dropped by the wayside until I stopped doing them all together. That, as it turned out, was not a good thing. You see, every time I coughed I peed. Every time I got out of a chair, I peed. Every time I walked across the room, I peed. It was a giant slide back to week one and a great disappointment to me as a person and a patient. I had let this happen. How could I let this happen? I was almost out of the diapers and now I am back in them and using two, three, four a day. At this point gluing my penis shut didn't seem like such a bad idea. This recovery is much tougher than I thought it was going to be. I thought I would have my prostate out and presto change-o I would be back to normal. I'm learning there is no back to normal with this thing, and the flu/bronchitis has shown me that. When you are recovering from prostate surgery you have to be diligent at all times. There are no two steps back because it's never just two steps back—it's like ten steps back. I am back to stage one of my recovery. I have set myself back three months and I have no one to blame but myself. I'm trying not to be too hard on myself. With my new attitude I am saying I made a mistake, so now I have to fix it. I am going to use my stupidity to warn others. I don't want anyone else to have to go through the set-back that I have gone through. Once you have the surgery, you are the doctor-on-duty twenty-four seven. You are responsible for your recovery. You can't let your guard down, and most important of all, you cannot stop doing the Kegel exercises. I have spoken!

The Saga of the Three-Month Appointment, Or Just Shoot Me Please

When I had my little flu set-back it occurred to me that maybe I should contact the doctor's office and let them know what was happening with me. Once again I emailed the office manager and said, "I've got the flu. I'm back up to five diapers a day. It's February and my next appointment isn't until May. I really think I should see the doctor sooner than May in case there is something wrong."

Within five minutes I got an email back, "How is March 21st at 10:20 a.m.?"

I grabbed the appointment and sat there looking at my computer screen. Why had she been able to get me an appointment two months earlier than the person who is responsible for making the doctor's follow up appointments? What power did the office manager have that the scheduler didn't have? This only reaffirmed a mantra that I have used my entire life and repeat over and over and over: "Let me speak to your supervisor. Let me speak to your supervisor. Let me speak to your supervisor." It's the only thing that works. The level-one people just don't have the power or the initiative to solve problems and find solutions. They are there to work their eight-hour day, get a paycheck, and play Words with Friends on their iPhone. If you are battling to recover from surgery or trying to get better theater seats or trying to get a defective washing machine fixed under warranty, "Let me speak to your supervisor," works every time. I pass this information on to you with the gratitude to my prostate and years of battling with morons in call centers in Calcutta or whatever the hell they call it now.

The Six-Month Visit... I Waited Six Months For This?

The saga of the three-month appointment has been long and hard. Because of illness and cancellations, it has stretched to the six-month appointment, but it was actually only five months since my surgery. It's like you take your car in for the 50,000 mile check up when it has 53,000 miles on it. If you are confused, go back and re-read the book. Just to refresh your memory, it went like this: they cancelled, then they cancelled again, then I cancelled, then they cancelled, and then I got the flu. It was easier for Trump to see Kim Jong-un than for me to get that next appointment which was supposed to be the three-month appointment but in actuality was a five-month appointment that they are calling the six-month appointment. Don't ask. Trying to do calculus is easier.

Needless to say, my mind was going full throttle the night before the appointment. My previous encounters with the office staff had not been good. Let's just say Netanyahu had a better relationship with Yasser Arafat. I was expecting to encounter the same experience—lots of lies and bombings. My mind was going a mile a minute. I had imagined the nurse coming in with a cold and distant attitude. I don't like cold and distant. I like warm and fuzzy, and cold and fuzzy would make me be angry. In my fantasy I had her talking rudely to me and me exploding in a tantrum, "How dare you talk to me like that! Do you know who I think I am??" I had built the meeting up in my mind to be the worst experience of my whole recovery, and I was prepared for that bitch of a nurse when I walked into the doctor's office.

She was out that day. Well, that was time well spent in my mind on nothing. Okay, so I have to readjust my fantasy; the tantrum will be about the time I had to wait to be seen by the doctor. I got there at 9:54 a.m. and those bastards made me wait until 9:56 a.m. So much for the "How long is it going to take?" tantrum. Don't you worry, in my fantasies I have a lot of bad things that could happen. Really bad things, things that could cause me to have a really big, loud, somebody get him a Valium tantrum. How about the time they keep me in the treatment room? Huh? How about that one? The nurse was in there to see me in literally three minutes. Come on people, work with me here. How the hell am I supposed to have a tantrum if you people are being so nice to me? Not Fair! To add to their niceness, this was a new nurse—a nurse who smiled, a nurse who asked how I was doing and how I was feeling. Now this bullshit is going to have to stop. You are ruining my big dramatic scene here.

The nurse takes the vitals and my blood pressure is 170/107. I don't feel tense. I'm not acting tense. Who knew that just thinking about having a tantrum could raise your blood pressure? The nurse was wonderful. She didn't say things like, "Wow! Somebody's head is gonna explode if you're not careful." She just asked if I had taken my medication or missed a dose or if there was something on my mind that was bothering me. You bet your ass there is. I want to have a tantrum and you people are treating me so nice that it's impossible to scream at anyone. That pressure is building up and my head's going to explode. This is all her fault.

The niceness continues. She told me to lie down and relax that someone would be in to see me soon. Okay, now I got it. This is where I'm left in the room for thirty minutes, forgotten like someone's taco from yesterday in the office kitchen. Okay, Tantrum 101 is about to begin.

Within four minutes a beautiful young women enters the room, "Hello, I'm Dr. [Whatever]. I'm the resident." Okay, now I know what's going on. The doctor is not going to see me. He's sending in his student doctors to do the dirty work, that tricky little bastard. However, this doctor was not so bad. There are people who can make an immediate connection, and this doctor was one of them. Beside that, she was efficient, intelligent and had a great bedside manner— but mostly she was caring, and I love caring. She was caring, and then out of the blue she asked about erectile dysfunction. Here I am talking about my hard-on—or lack thereof—with a complete stranger doctor lady. This could possibly be a tantrum moment. This could be a great tantrum moment, "I can't discuss this with you. You're a lady; you don't have a dick. I need to talk about erectile dysfunction to someone with a dick, you know, man to man, with a guy who knows what it feels like to be limp like a plate of over-cooked spaghetti." That scene wasn't going to happen, how could I have a tantrum with someone who actually cared if I ever got laid again? She was wonderful and we finished the interview without me doing the death scene from Hamlet or pointing my finger in anger and demanding to see her supervisor. I was a good boy. I did timidly ask, "Will I be seeing the doctor at today's visit?" Now, you know I was just waiting for the wrong answer, an answer to give me an excuse to have one huge temper tantrum right there in the treatment room. In my mind, that would mean I am not important enough to be seen by the big guy and the entire office would know that when I had my tantrum.

She smiled and said, "Of course you will see the doctor. I'm just getting all the details down so he can spend more time with you." Good answer! She leaves me alone in the room, letting me know the doctor will be with me soon. I can hear the doctor in the next examination room talking to another patient. My first thought, *Are you two timing me? Are you seeing other patients?* You know, like we're dating. Then I pondered, why do they make the walls so thin in those examining rooms? Do I have to hear that this other guy's prostate is the size of a grapefruit? Do I need this information? They spend millions of dollars on the hospital building and then use tissue paper to divide the examining rooms. I can hear the patient asking all kinds of questions. As a matter of fact, he asked some of the same questions I was going to ask, and I heard the doctor's answer. Maybe the hospitals are on to something here. Save time answering questions with thin walls. Now my fear is that this patient is going to take up more time and ask the doctor to read chapters from his medical journal, the entire section on erectile dysfunction, and then re-enact the day he cut up his first cadaver. He's going be there forever. He's gonna miss the fall football season because of this guy. He's gonna the re-release of Star Wars. He gonna miss…. Wait. Suddenly the other room goes silent. I know what's happened, the patient has coded and they are bringing in the crash cart. Lo and behold, there is a tap on the door. Why do they always tap? What do they think we're doing in there while we wait; going through their bandage drawer? Anyway, it's the doctor and he looks more relaxed than I remember him. Maybe it's because he has my prostate in a jar sitting on the shelf at Cedar's research center? He seemed more relaxed and less nervous. Or maybe it was that I was more relaxed and less nervous. Who knows, this is the first time I've dated this guy.

We had a wonderful chat. I asked him if the cancer could come back, and to my surprise he told me it could. If one cell had gone to my bladder or bone we could have another round of cancer. This was not what I wanted to hear or what I expected to hear. I thought I was cured, but with cancer you are never really cured. It hangs over your head like Marie Antoinette's executioner's blade. He then tagged the subject by saying that the chances of a reoccurrence happening in my case were about 5%. That certainly gave Madame Antoinette a new lease on life because it meant that there was a 95% chance that it would not come back. I'll take those odds. I was greatly relieved, but with me I'm never really completely relieved. I'll be worried about this cancer until they close the lid on my casket, and probably two weeks after that.

We discussed all kinds of things. I showed him my Kegel App for my iPhone and he explained to me how important it was for me to continue to do the Kegels. I used to have two muscles in my groin and now I have only one. I have to strengthen the one measly muscle I have left to prevent myself from pissing my pants while at the Opera or waiting in line at Burger King. I listened long and hard and I got his message. I began doing Kegels as soon as I got into the car. A house doesn't have to fall on me. If I want to get better I have to participate. My friend Bob Benjamin has been my Kegel coach. He'll email me twice a day, "Did you do your Kegels?" It's a wonderful thing to have someone care and have someone remind you that you have to care about yourself to get better. "DO YOUR KEGELS" will be my next tattoo. My only tattoo. I'm not getting a tattoo, who am I kidding? I cry when I have to get a flu shot. Do you really think I'm going to sit there while they puncture my arm twelve thousand times—and in colored ink?

Then without warning, the conversations takes a whole new direction and the doctor began talking about erections. Why is everyone so interested in my erections? I'm not even that interested in them. Everyone in this office is obsessed with my erections. Can't they just let me figure this out by myself? He casually asked if I had had any erections lately. It's a sentence I never thought I would ever hear from a doctor. The strange thing is, every guy who has had this surgery has called me to tell me about his erection. I have heard things that I never wanted to hear from people I'm not that close to, nor plan to be. I certainly never thought that I would answer the erection question so easily with, "I had half a one last week." The doctor was thrilled. He told me I was way ahead of the rest. If this were the Boy Scouts I could have gotten a merit badge for erections.

Then the conversation got even weirder for me. He started telling me that there is now a generic Viagra that it only costs one dollar a pill. Right away I'm thinking, *erections are on sale?* What a country we live in. The doctor told me how and when to take Viagra and to try it out before actually having sex. You know, a test flight. "Masturbate," he said, "See how it goes." Oh my God, the doctor just gave me permission to masturbate. I asked him if he wanted me to do try now and did he have any dirty magazines. No laugh. This visit is turning out a lot better than I ever imagined. You'll get no tantrum from me here on this point.

We spoke about all kinds of things. I told him I was writing a book about my experience and he told me of a doctor who had gone through prostate cancer and also wrote a book, but his book was too clinical and he couldn't figure out what the market would be for it. I told him mine had comical elements and touched on my innermost thoughts. He thought it was a great idea to add comedy to the cancer (is this getting as weird for you as it was for me?).

The surprise part of the visit came when he told me he wanted to see me in six months and that I would need PSA tests every six months for the next few years. You see, with cancer you are never really left alone. They are always checking on you to see if the little bastard has come back again. It's like you get cancer and then have a dark cloud hanging over you for the rest of your life. Nothing you can do but accept your fate and move on, and that's what I'm planning on doing. I'm going to enjoy the years I have left. I have spent my whole life worrying about being ill, and to what end? I got ill and there was nothing I could do about it but deal with it. That's the best course of action for anyone in this situation. Enjoy each day of your life, because you don't know when it will be your last. Look at those people who are killed in their home when a plane crashes into it. They weren't even going on a trip and they are killed in a plane crash. When your time is up, your time is up, and you have no control over it. The best advice I can give you is live and enjoy your life. Worry will fix nothing—but do your Kegels.

There was one last bit of business. I had to give a urine specimen before I left the office. The nurse takes me into the bathroom and says, "Have you ever given a urine specimen before?" and I'm thinking, *What kind of moron do you think I am?* "Because this is a little different," she continues. She shows me something that looks like a spittoon sitting two feet off the floor. "You pee in this," she says.

"You're shitting me," I reply.

"Please don't do that... just pee in there."

Everyone has a sense of humor. She exits and I look into the spittoon. At the bottom is this spinning wheel thingy that I have to pee into. I am a little hesitant because I think when I pee into it, it's going to spray all over the place, but it doesn't. I see the spinning wheel and I see my pee go down to never been seen again. So long fella, we had a good run. Then all of a sudden there is a printer on the shelf and it starts printing out all kind of data. I get hysterical laughing. Pee in here, read it there. When I'm done, the nurse comes in and takes the paper to show the doctor. I then have an ultra sound of my bladder, and I'm good to go. It's like I'm in the middle of some science fiction movie, *It Peed From Outer Space.*

After he had looked at all the tests, he tells me I was good. The doctor and I shook hands. He told me he was happy with my progress. We will meet again in six months and I will tell him about my erections, or lack there of. Maybe I should start an erection journal. Could be interesting, "On Tuesday I had a stiffy when I got on a crowded bus and was pushed into an anxiety support dog." It's not necessary to write the journal. I'll come for my visits, he will tell me the results of my latest PSA test, and I'll see him again in another six months. It's my new relationship. I guess, better with him than the guy at Forrest Lawn.

As I was leaving, the receptionist stopped me to give me my appointment for six months from now. In my head I'm thinking, *This will never happen. They will change the appointment five times before I get to see the doctor again,* but I said not a word. I just entered the info into my iPhone calendar and took the orders for the next PSA test. I was even smiling as I did it. So much has changed in me over the last five months. I have learned so much and come so far. Cancer is a life changing experience. It makes you stop and think. It makes you reevaluate. It makes you different. I still have a long way to go, but at least I know where I'm headed now. I have a plan of attack. I have an end plan. Wait. That's a bad choice of words. I have a goal. Yes, much better.

I took the information packet from the receptionist, put it in my briefcase/diaper bag, and as I walked out the door I thought to myself, *Did I forget anything?* The only thing I could think of was, *I forgot to have a tantrum.* Change is good.

Epilogue... Not the End, But the Beginning

That's it? This is the end of the adventure? I lose my prostate and I'm in diapers for the rest of my life? This is the dream ending I've been writing about for the last five months? No. That's not what I've been writing about for the last five months. It's just one of the facets of this surgery you have to deal with in recovery. Losing my prostate to cancer was just the first step in an adventure, one in which I learned so much about myself that it wasn't even funny. I just made it funny. I learned things, like that I could be grateful to cancer for what it has taught me. Grateful to cancer, there's a phrase you will not read in any other book. Who is grateful to cancer? What idiot would be grateful to cancer? I guess the answer is I would.

Let's take some of the things I learned over the last five months, for instance. Things like finding out how much I am loved. Who knew? I certainly didn't know. I had no idea that my friends would rally around me like an army of love. How could I have known? I was always told I was unlovable, but cancer and my friends have taught me otherwise. Remember that day I was sitting in my bedroom and burst into tears in gratitude? That is when the realization hit me. I guess it was like when Madame Currie found radium. The joy of the discovery after all those years of hard work must have been overwhelming, so she cried. That's how it was with me. I got it. I finally got it. I am loved because I am a good person. Now that's not to say I'm "cured" of my insanities. I will always carry them with me like a badge of courage. Hester Prynne had her scarlet "A". I carry my navy blue "I" for insecurity and insanity. It took me many years to get this way; I'm not going to be fixed overnight. What I have been given over these last five months is the knowledge that my thinking has been all wrong. I cannot deny the eye-opening experience that was given to me during my recuperation. I cannot deny that people didn't come around to share love with me because I was a bad person. They came around because they were returning the love that I had given to them over the years. I cannot thank them enough, those wonderful people who took the time to teach me this lesson.

Then there was the lesson of gratitude. I have an angel who sits on my shoulder. I honestly believe that I carry with me a guardian angel. It was he who made me ask for my doctor to take a second PSA test. I had taken one and the results were 4.8. Six months later I asked for another and he agreed. Those results were 6.5. I have never done that in all the years that I have been taking that test. Why did I do it now? I have no idea, and my only answer is that my guardian angel had me covered. I am the luckiest man on earth to be blessed with a guardian angel, and I don't care who thinks I'm crazy for believing I have one. I even know his name, Gary Weinberg. He was my agent and we were closer than brothers. I believe the doctors found this cancer in the first six months of its development, and I have Gary to thank for that. Thank you my angel! We got it when it was easily remove. Ha! Easily removed. Did you see what I just said there? Easily removed, yeah, easy like removing senior citizens from the all-you-can-eat buffet table at five p.m. It was not easily removed, it was the most difficult thing I ever had to go through in my life. Yet, I made it through.

That's another lesson I learned on this cancer journey. You can get through anything if you just take it one day at a time and keep positive. A positive attitude is the most important thing you can carry with you when battling cancer. I believe in endorphins. I believe they fight along with you and that positive attitude is your best endorphin creator. I was lucky enough to have that positive attitude. It may have been from sheer stupidity. I had no idea what I was about to go through or what the end results would be, so I laughed and joked and looked for the silver lining in everything that happened to me—with the exception of making those goddamn office visits. I had good role models. I had friends who battled stage four cancer with a smile on their face and are still here to tell us about it. I have a friend with a heart transplant and another with a heart *and* liver transplant who wrote comedy all through the time he was stuck in the hospital. There is something to that positive attitude, and I suggest you use it if you are ever faced with an episode of cancer or cancelled airplane flights or bad service in a restaurant or, well, life.

I want anyone who has gone through prostate cancer to read this book and know there is a tomorrow. I want them to know that there is hope. I want them to know that, sure, it's not easy to fight this fight, but it is doable. Listen, if I can do this, you can too. I didn't ask to get cancer. It wasn't on my bucket list, but I got it despite the fact that I had worried about getting cancer since I was in the sixth grade. Oh yes, I distinctly remember feeling a lump in my earlobe and knowing that I had developed the deadly earlobe cancer. When I told Miss Prichard I needed to see the nurse because I thought I had cancer, the expression on her face was burned into my memory banks. It was a cross between laughter and pity. How does a child in the sixth grade develop a fear of cancer? What can be done to a sixth grader to make them fearful for their health? I know the answers now. My parents' lack of caring instilled in me a fear of dying that I carried with me my entire life. When an illness finally came, even I was surprised at how well I reacted. I reacted like an adult with a serious medical condition. How absolutely refreshing is that? There are shrinks all over this country who are taking credit for this accomplishment, and probably rightly so.

Trust. Through the entire experience I never once mentioned the word trust. That's because I trust no one. I know that if it's at all possible, I will be disappointed by anyone who is close to me. I had learned as a child that those closest to me would be the first to let me down, and those let-downs would be the most painful. It's why I'm so goddamn self-sufficient. I depend on no one and I'm never disappointed. Oh trust me, I let my guard down now and then, and people prove me right. They disappoint me. It's after one of those episodes that I crawl back into my cocoon of safety and shut myself off from the world. I have adopted the philosophy of expect nothing and you will never be disappointed. Yet here I was with my life totally out of my control asking myself to trust those around me to take care of me. I, who watches the barber as she cuts every hair, now had to give up control of the direction of my life. I had to trust the doctor knew what he was doing. I had to trust the nurses would take care of me. I had to trust that I would make it through this medical episode like a shining star like my Facebook friend, Dot McQuisten, says I am. Me, a shining star? No way. How could I be? Trust was never on my registry of positive traits. I was not good at trusting others, so how could I trust that Dot was right or that anything through this whole ordeal would turn out to my liking? There I was with my life in the hands of hundreds of people who I was forced to trust. I had to do the biggest surrender I ever had to do. I had to trust—and look how it all turned out. The cancer is removed and I'm here to bitch about the goddamn diapers.

I don't want you to think my life is all rosy and that it's all sunshine and lollipops after the surgery. It's not. It's hard. It's hard to worry that you may smell or that your pants are wet. It's hard to be forced to carry extra supplies with you everywhere you go. It's hard to suddenly realize you are not the person you were before the surgery. It's hard to realize that you have aged and that this is what happens to men as they get older. It's just hard (but not where you want it hard). There is not a day that goes by that I do not feel sorry for myself for three minutes every morning. There is not a time when I don't say, "When will this incontinence end?" There just isn't a time when I don't wish I had my old life back, but I am also so grateful that I am here, that I have been given a second chance, and that for today I am cancer free.

If there is anything I want you take away from my experience, it's how grateful I am to be alive. I want you to know that if you are about to go through prostate cancer or if you have gone through prostate cancer, you are not alone. I want you to know that we are all in this together, every man who has ever had to have this surgery. Most of all, I want you to know that we care. I care. Thousands of people out there care. You are not alone. There is nothing to be ashamed of. You have done nothing wrong but get older and get prostate cancer. Hold your head high and begin the battle a winner.

Let me leave you with this: my prostate cancer has been the biggest and best learning experience of my life. It has taught me about love and life and trust and surrender and love. Mostly it has taught me about love. If you're feeling a little low because you have had prostate cancer, pick up those diapers and face the world, because you have the rest of your life to get back in order. You are not a victim. You are a winner. Now go out there and win!!!

Peace.

The Epilogue to the Epilogue

I bet you thought we were done. I'll bet you thought we were all going to live in a big show in Never-Never Land. I'll bet you thought everything was going to be peachy keen and we would ride off into the sunset together. I'll bet you wanted a happy ending. Well, guess again. Don't you know you are never done with cancer? You think you're done but cancer has a whole different take on the subject. It needs to torment you and drag out the recovery so that it will weaken your resolve. You must never let it weaken your resolve because if you do, cancer wins. Here's what happened.

Everything was going along just hunky-dory. I was feeling fine, the diaper usage was back down to one a day, the energy was coming back, and the body was building itself back up. I could see the light at the end of the tunnel. As they say, "Who knew the light at the end of the tunnel was a train?"

I got up to pee at 6 a.m. I had been doing it all along. Nothing to worry about. It was just my morning pee—we all do it. Everything was working like it should and I happened to look down. The bathroom was dark, but even in the darkness I could tell something wasn't right. I turned on the light only to see a toilet bowl filled with blood. Now I'm not doctor, but I knew this was not normal. I ran to the phone to call the doctor, it's 6 a.m., there is no one in the medical profession at 6 a.m. My God, the golf courses don't even open until ten. I sent

117

my doctor an email and sat down in the living room to have a massive anxiety attack, because in my mind I was dying. It was a nice anxiety attack too. It was the kind of anxiety attack where you feel yourself falling away, like you're falling off a cliff and there is nothing you can do to stop you from falling into the row of spikes at the end of the fall. I couldn't breathe. My arms went numb. It was the most horrible hour of my life, and I've had some pretty horrible hours.

Soon I got an email back from the doctor, "Nothing to worry about. It's normal. Come to see me in the next two weeks." Yeah, like I'm going to let this ride for another two weeks.

I called his office at 9:01 a.m., "The doctor wants to see me immediately."

I don't think the girl had even finished her donut when I called, "Well, he can see you in two weeks. Is that good?"

"Let me put it to you this way, if you got up and saw a toilet bowl full of blood would it be good with you??"

"Oh. How is tomorrow at 9 a.m.?"

"Perfect."

I guess they're beginning to understand me better.

The next morning I was there bright and early. I was up at 4 a.m., and I paced around the house like a caged tiger. I was trying to calm myself down, but when faced with a bowl of blood, my only answer was "the cancer has spread." 9:00 a.m. never came, or at least it felt like it would never come. I got in to see the doctor right on time and he said the only thing I was not   prepared for, "I need to do a cystoscopy." Another cystoscopy? No! I couldn't. I just couldn't. There is no way I'm going through that again. You cannot do a cystoscopy on me today. I am not emotionally ready to do that. No. I won't do it.

As I lay on the table about to have a cystoscopy, the nurse is holding my foot to comfort me. Hello, I have hands. She was gently rubbing my foot as the doctor said, "There is something in your bladder. It could be a tumor, but it could also be scar tissue from the surgery."

"What else could it be? Maybe damage from 14 cystoscopies?"

He needed to do a biopsy under general anesthesia tomorrow at 5 a.m. Another surgery, another hospital stay, another "May I see your photo I.D.?" because lord knows there are a gang of roving thieves who are out there stealing bladder biopsies.

It's the whole scene all over again. The happy nurse. The blood taker. The anesthesiologist who is so peppy and happy and full of charm and life that you want to slap her across the face with a bedpan. It was the whole scene from the original surgery, and I hated every minute of it. I hated that my body had put me back in this position. I hated the lack of control I had over my life. I hated that possibly this could be the end of my life as I knew it.

The nurse got me all ready for the surgery. This time I remember going into the operating room. This time I remember climbing onto the table. This time I remember saying, "Here we go," as I could feel the anesthesia working its way through my system.

When I opened my eyes, it was about an hour later. I was groggy and in no pain. My best friend, Ben Blake, was there to take me home. I didn't see the doctor. I didn't see anyone but the charge nurse who told me it was okay to leave. I fled that place like the Jews left Egypt with Moses. Only I didn't wander for forty years. I went right home and crawled into bed.

I had Ben stop at the pharmacy to pick up my prescription for antibiotics. Horse pills again. I took the pills. I flushed them down with something akin to the Atlantic Ocean. The next morning I sat in the living room. Waiting. No pain. Feeling nothing but anxiety waiting for the doctor's call. It was a Friday. If I didn't get the call today, I would have to wait for the weekend, and the thought of waiting two more days had my anxiety on a level ten. At about 6 p.m. the phone rang. I saw the caller I.D. It was Cedars. I picked up the phone just as cheery as I could possibly be.

"Hello, Steve, Dr. Kim. It's benign. Looks like it is scar tissue, which looks very much like a tumor, but it's not. So we're good to go."

Needless to say I was over the moon. The anxiety left me and was replaced with tears of joy. The release you get when you learn that you have beat cancer yet again is beyond description. It's nirvana.

I was a very good patient. I finished taking the antibiotics and thought I was over the worst of this ordeal, when suddenly I began urinating at an alarming rate. It went on for a day. I convinced myself it was just the side affects of the biopsy, but every time I went to urinate, I was in pain.

After about three days of this I emailed the doctor, "I'm sorry to bother you but...blah blah blah." Looks like I picked up a urinary tract infection. I was prescribed another ten days of horse pills. At this point I could be entered in the Kentucky Derby. It took the full ten days for the infection to leave. Even when the pills had all been taken I felt myself getting ill again—despite the fact that I was not. The mind is an incredible organ and makes your body do truly strange things.

It took a full two weeks before the constant urination and pain ended. It did end. It was over. The whole episode was over. They never found out where the blood came from. I had a full MRI, and everything was normal. It was just one of those things. One of those things that only happens to me! A blood vessel burst or a stitch opened or...who knows? At this point, I don't care. It wasn't cancer. That's all that matters.

This whole episode set my recovery back about two months. I began changing diapers regularly like a two year-old does, but I was finally feeling better and getting back to my old self—and I do mean old. I have aged incredibly over the last six months. I never had a grey hair on my head. Suddenly I have grey sideburns. Hello Grecian Formula! I have never felt the ravages of time, but this little episode has taught me that I am old and I have to get used to it.

What have I learned over the last six months? Never take your time on this earth for granted. You may be on the road to recovery, but that road has potholes and detours and traffic jams. Think of your recovery as the 405 Freeway. It's the Fourth of July at 7 p.m., there's a car on fire in the number three lane, and you just got a flat tire. The only thing that's not happening is a slow speed chase. In other words, your recovery is never easy. It's never what you plan, and it's never the end of a medical episode. It's a continuing saga with you as the star. There's a line in a Sondheim song, "Life isn't easy." Nothing could be truer. Life is not easy. I learned that this year. Troubles come and troubles go, but they are never over. You just have to handle each episode as it comes along. You just have to deal with everything one day at a time. You just have to surrender your will, because all the worry and anxiety and fear and what-ifs will not do you any good. It's out of your hands. It's a big surrender when you are fighting cancer. There are no set rules. There is no promised outcome. It just is what it is.

I am very grateful for the wonderful friends that carried me through this whole ordeal. I don't know what I would have done without them. I am also grateful for my sense of humor, which has kept me going and gave me something to write about. I want to say this is the end of this book. I want to say there won't be an epilogue to the epilogue's epilogue, but I can't. I don't know what the future holds. I just know today. Today I can say… it's the end.

And now, if you'll excuse me, I'm going to change my diaper.

Bye-bye!

CPSIA information can be obtained
at www.ICGtesting.com
Printed in the USA
FSHW021249051119
63782FS

9 781629 334929